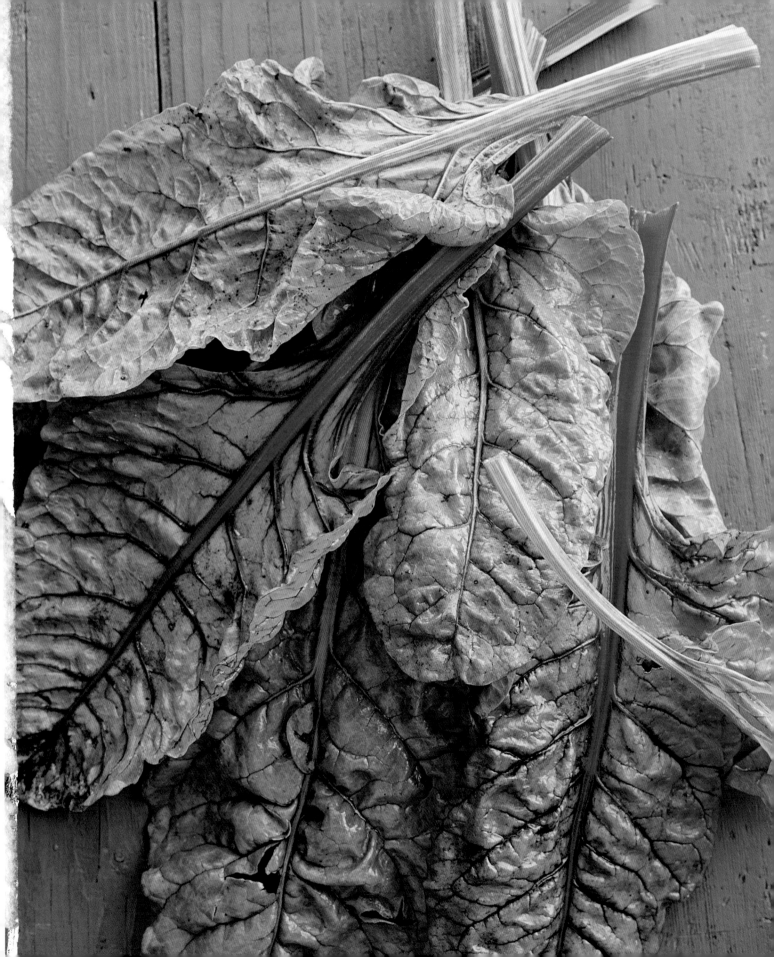

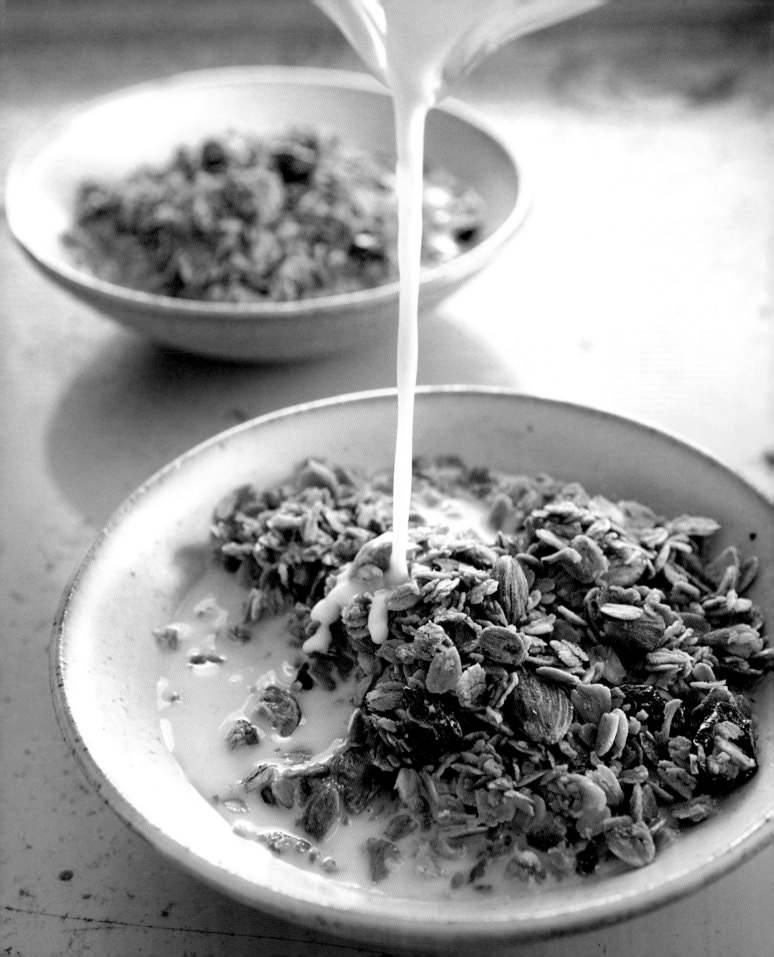

healthy in a hurry

text
Karen Ansel, MS, RD

recipes
Charity Ferreira

photographs
Maren Caruso

weldon**owen**

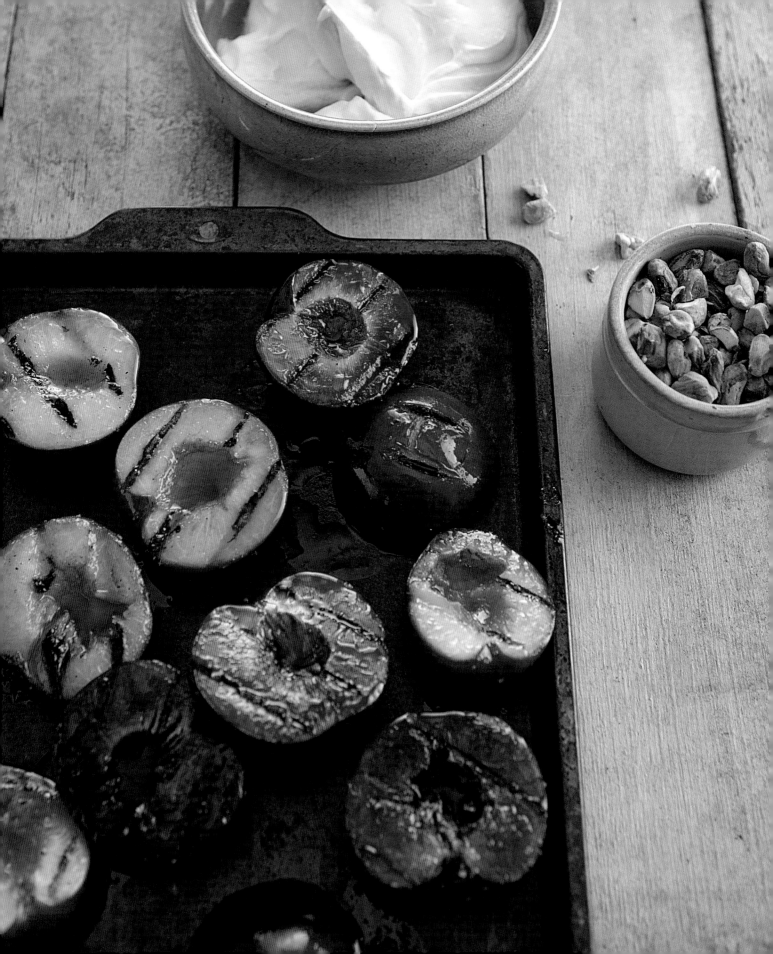

CONTENTS

You don't need to spend your time wading through all the nutritional advice that's out there—much of it conflicting—in order to live a healthy lifestyle. As a busy nutritionist, I've discovered that there are just two important tricks to getting delicious, healthy meals on the table, and knowing them will simplify your life and reduce stress around eating well, especially with a packed schedule. The first is choosing lots of fresh, unprocessed foods, and the second is having a foolproof plan to get you in and out of the kitchen quickly. This book delivers on both.

"This book is filled with easy-to-follow advice that simplifies the essentials of healthy eating."

Healthy in a Hurry is your road map for creating quick, nourishing meals from wholesome ingredients. It's filled with easy-to-follow advice and useful nutritional information that simplify the essentials of healthy eating. Loaded with flavor-packed recipes from talented cookbook author Charity Ferreira, it will show you, step by step, how to prepare tasty, satisfying food without spending hours in the kitchen. You'll feast on sweet fruit smoothies, tender whole-grain muffins, refreshing salads, comforting soups, hearty proteins, enticing vegetable and grain sides, and more. And because a healthy diet should always leave room for a little indulgence, you'll also find recipes for savory snacks and decadent desserts.

So what are you waiting for—it's time to get cooking!

Karen Ansel

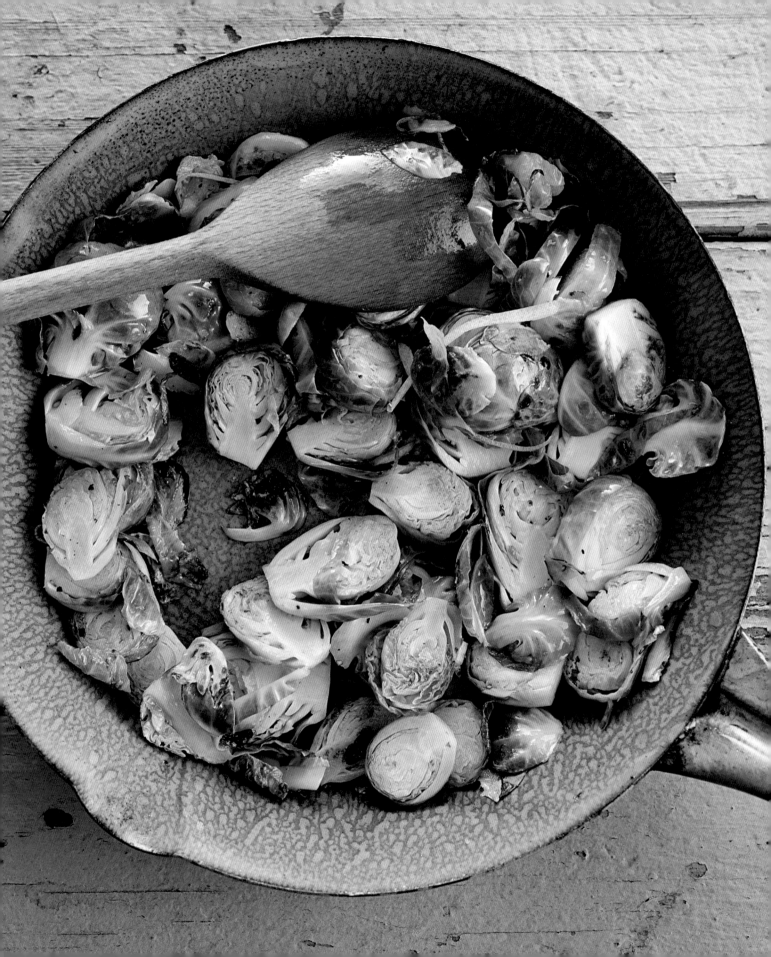

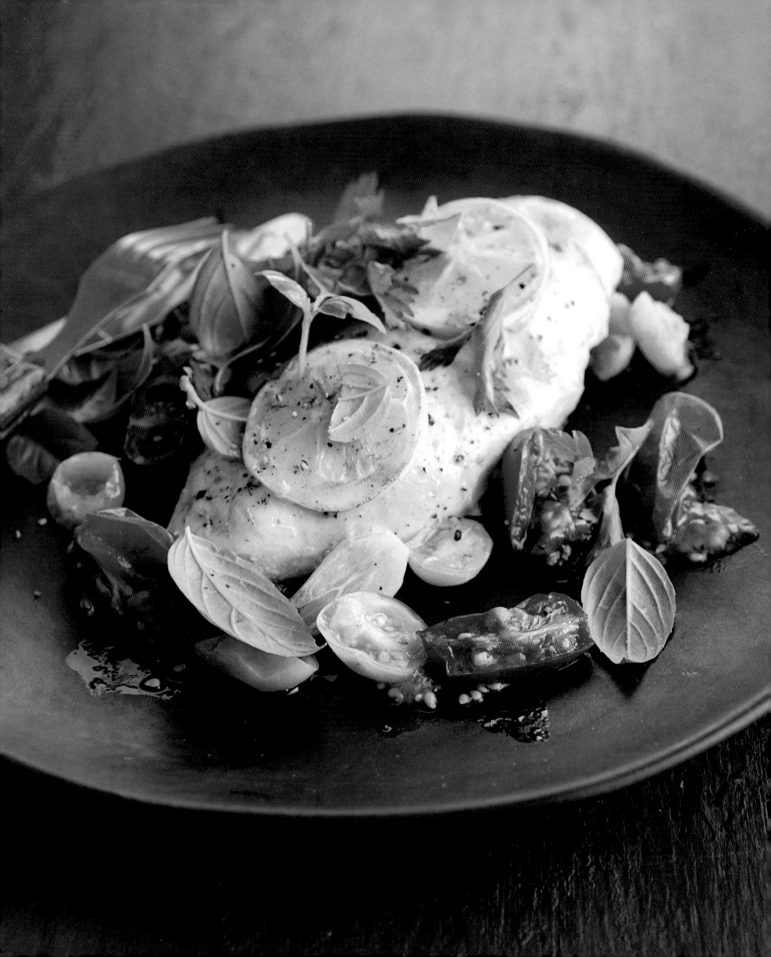

With ever-changing food trends, eating right in today's world can seem complicated. But it doesn't have to be. Remember these six simple steps, and aim for a wide variety of fresh, wholesome foods for optimal health and energy.

EATING HEALTHY EVERY DAY

STAY FLEXIBLE

Each of us has unique nutritional needs depending on our age, gender, and activity level. Most women require between 1,800 and 2,000 calories a day, while men can usually eat a little more, from 2,200 to 2,600 calories.

PUT COLOR ON YOUR PLATE

Fruits and vegetables are brimming with disease-preventing vitamins, minerals, plant chemicals, and fiber, so strive to fill at least half of your plate with produce, and go for as many colors as you can. The more hues your produce contains, the more nutrition it packs. Balance the remainder of your plate with one-fourth whole grains and one-fourth lean protein.

KEEP FATS HEALTHY

It's fine to eat up to a third of your daily calories from fat, provided it's from healthful sources like avocados; nuts and seeds; olives; and olive, peanut, and canola oils. Depending on your size and how active you are, a healthful range of fat is 40 to 75 grams for most women and 50 to 100 grams for most men.

Try to avoid hydrogenated and trans fats entirely and limit saturated fat found in butter, fatty cuts of red meat, poultry with skin, and full-fat dairy products. Limit cholesterol, another type of fat found exclusively in animal products, to 200 to 300 milligrams a day.

DO GRAINS RIGHT

Roughly half of our calories should come from carbohydrates, to supply the energy our bodies and brains need to thrive. Women should aim for between 225 to 250 grams of carbohydrates per day, while men will require between 275 and 325 grams.

Like fat, not all carbohydrates are created equal. Choosing minimally processed, fiber-rich carbohydrates from whole grains such as oats, quinoa, and whole-wheat bread, pasta, and couscous provides sustained energy to keep you feeling your best. Eating these, along with plenty of fruits, vegetables, and beans, will provide the 25 to 28 grams of fiber needed to keep us full and promote digestive and heart health.

THINK LEAN PROTEIN

Slowly digested protein helps us stay full, keeps our immune systems strong, and builds muscle, tissues, and hormones. Yet we need surprisingly little—only 10 to 20 percent of our daily calories. That's roughly 45 to 100 grams for women and 55 to 130 grams for men. To minimize harmful saturated fats hidden in many protein foods, opt for lean sources of fat such as 1 percent or nonfat milk, beans, tofu, fish, lean meats, and skinless poultry.

GO EASY ON THE SALT

Most of the sodium in our diets comes from packaged foods. Eating too many of these can quickly add up, exceeding the 1,500 to 2,300 milligram upper limit that most of us should have each day. Start with fresh foods and you'll naturally reduce the amount of sodium in your diet. When buying packaged foods, compare brands and look closely at the sodium content. And don't be afraid to try low salt versions—you'll be pleasantly surprised.

Planning healthy meals is a balancing act. Offset a hearty breakfast with a light lunch—or snack on fresh fruit if you'll be enjoying a substantial dinner. Regardless of what your main dish is, be sure to round out your plate with plenty of nutrient-rich fruits and vegetables.

CREATING BALANCED MEALS

A WEEK'S WORTH OF HEALTHY EATING

	breakfast	lunch	dinner	snack
monday	Egg sandwich; vegetable juice	Quinoa salad; butternut squash soup	Salmon tacos; black beans	Fresh fruit
tuesday	Granola with 1% milk and fresh berries	Turkey wrap; carrot slaw	Soba noodle bowl; spinach salad	Guacamole with baked tortilla chips
wednesday	Farina or oatmeal with fresh fruit	Black bean burger; sweet potato fries	Steak and arugula salad; tabbouleh	Yogurt dip with crudités
thursday	Fruit smoothie; whole-wheat toast	Greek chicken salad; gazpacho	Whole-wheat flatbread with turkey sausage; roasted asparagus	Fruit and nut bar
friday	Tofu scramble; fruit juice	Portobello mushroom sandwich; roasted broccoli	Steamed fish with vegetables; whole-wheat couscous	Ricotta and vegetable crostini
saturday	Pancakes; sliced fresh fruit	Salad with tuna and white beans	Pork stir-fry with vegetables and brown rice	Kale chips
sunday	Vegetable hash and poached egg	Bean quesadilla with fruit salsa	Seafood stew with quinoa; sautéed green beans	Hummus and baby carrots

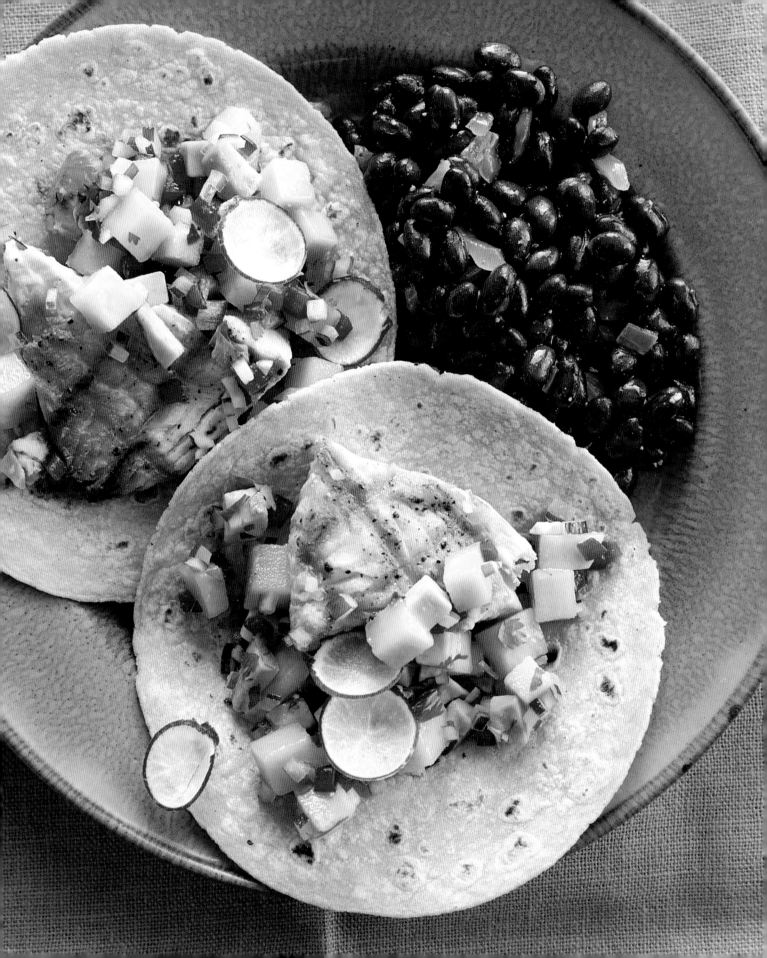

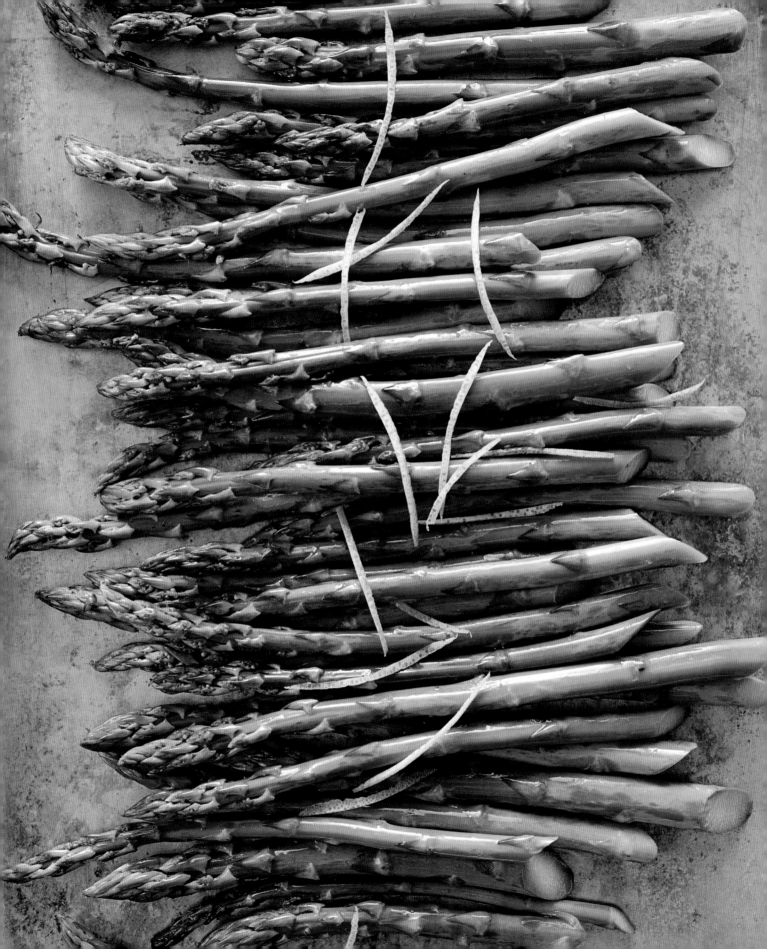

Recognizing the impact that foods have on our overall health and well-being is the first step in eating well, but putting that knowledge into action can sometimes be a challenge. Here are a handful of simple ways to enjoy nutritious meals on a hectic schedule.

KEYS TO SUCCESS

SHOP AND COOK ON THE WEEKENDS

If you have a busy week ahead, you'll be amazed at what a few hours of prep work on the weekend will do to reduce stress and improve your meals during the week: cook a big batch of brown rice or beans; wash and chop lettuce and vegetables as soon as you get home from the market; hard-boil eggs for salads and sandwiches; premake a pasta sauce, like pesto or tomato sauce, and store it in the freezer. If your weekend is just as busy, consider buying shortcut foods, like precut vegetables, prewashed greens, and premade spreads or sauces.

STOCK YOUR PANTRY WITH WHOLESOME FOODS

A well-stocked pantry—from flavor boosters like oils, vinegars, and spices to complex carbohydrates like beans, brown rice, and whole-wheat pasta—takes the stress out of meal planning and prep because it ensures that you have the basics to throw together a fantastic meal even if you are too busy to get to the store. Turn to page 210 for a full list of suggested pantry items.

EMBRACE LEFTOVERS

Making extra food to store means having a premade meal for your lunch bag, or a home-cooked dinner waiting for you after a busy day. Most cooked leftovers will keep in an airtight container in the refrigerator for about 4 days, or in the freezer for 3–4 months; let the food cool completely before you pack it up for storage. Freeze liquid-based meals like soups and stews in small batches so you can heat up just enough for one or two servings, and clearly label items for freezing. Thaw frozen foods in the refrigerator or microwave, never at room temperature.

COOK WITH THE SEASONS

Whether you're shopping at a grocery store, local market, or farmers' market, try to seek out produce that you know is in season. Produce tastes best when it's at its peak; plus, it's likely to be more nutritious, because the longer produce sits in a truck in transit, the more nutrients it loses. Turn to page 212 for more information on when to buy seasonal produce.

SHOPPING SMARTS
A trip to the grocery store doesn't have to be an overwhelming experience if you add some strategy to your shopping routine.

make a list A shopping list will save you time and stress at the store. If you can, organize your list by food category to save even more time, and to keep you from having to double back through the aisles.

keep it simple Focus on fresh foods, which are most often found along the perimeter of a grocery store. When you're shopping within the aisles, look for unprocessed or minimally processed foods without a lot of added ingredients. Choose all-natural, low-sodium versions of canned foods when available.

be flexible Don't be afraid to make substitutions if the item on your list is not available or not in season. Push yourself to try new foods so you don't get stuck in a rut!

Making a point to incorporate nutrient-rich foods into your diet is a smart way to approach shopping and meal planning. The recipes in this book highlight the following superfoods, so you can reach for the most beneficial ingredients the next time you're at the market.

A GUIDE TO SUPERFOODS

APPLES

Buying Look for firm fruit with smooth skin free of bruises and blemishes. Buy organic when possible, as conventional apples tend to have high levels of pesticides.

Storing Let ripen at room temperature; apples will keep in the refrigerator for up to 2 months.

Healthy tip Don't peel that apple! The skin of an apple contains much of its healthful nutrients, including fiber and powerful antioxidants that may fight cancer.

Using Enjoy apples on their own, or slice and add to salads. Tart apples are ideal for making crisps and applesauce.

ARTICHOKES

Buying Look for firm, heavy, medium-sized artichokes. To test for freshness, squeeze the artichoke; it should squeak.

Storing Refrigerate in a plastic bag in the crisper for up to 5 days.

Quick tip Baby artichokes will cook faster than regular artichokes and are not as time-consuming to trim. To save even more time, buy all-natural precooked frozen or canned artichokes.

Using Steaming is a classic way to prepare artichokes. They can also be grilled, baked, and even shaved and served raw in salads.

ASPARAGUS

Buying Choose firm stalks with tightly closed heads. Avoid asparagus with slimy tips or thick, woody stalks.

Storing Place in a plastic bag in the crisper, or stand stalks upright in a small amount of water and cover with a plastic bag; refrigerate for up to 4 days.

Prep tip Instead of cutting the base off, hold the stalk loosely and snap off the bottom. The stalk will break where it starts to get tough.

Using Sauté, steam, roast, or grill asparagus and serve as a side; blanch and add to salads or pastas.

AVOCADOS

Buying Choose avocados that are heavy and blemish-free. If you plan on eating it right away, choose an avocado that is slightly soft and yields to gentle pressure.

Storing Let ripen at cool room temperature. Once ripe, store in the refrigerator for up to 2 days.

Prep tip Avocado flesh browns quickly, so don't cut an avocado until just before using. Lemon or lime juice will help prevent discoloration.

Using Slice or chop avocados for salads, sandwiches, wraps, and salsas; mash for dips and spreads.

BANANAS

Buying Choose bananas based on when you want to eat them: those with green coloration will need a few days to ripen, whereas yellow bananas with brown flecks should be eaten within a day or two.

Storing Let ripen at cool room temperature. Ripe bananas can be stored in the refrigerator, but the skins will blacken.

Quick tip To hasten the ripening of a banana, place it in a paper bag with an apple.

Using Peel and eat bananas out of hand, or slice and eat with low-fat or nonfat yogurt or milk and cereal; add to smoothies and baked goods.

BEANS (DRIED)

Includes black beans, chickpeas, kidney beans, lentils, lima beans, pinto beans, white beans

Buying Buy dried beans in bulk from a store that has a good product turnover. If buying canned beans, choose low-sodium or no-sodium-added varieties.

Storing Store dried beans in a cool, dry place for up to 1 year. Cooked beans can be stored in an airtight container or plastic bag in the refrigerator for up to 3 days or in the freezer for up to 3 months.

Healthy tip Get in the habit of cooking a large batch of beans on the weekend and freezing it (drain and cool beans before storing). You will have more options if you buy dried beans, and they will be more flavorful and lower in sodium than canned beans.

Using Purée beans for dips and spreads; add to soups and salads; flavor with herbs and spices and serve as a simple side.

BEETS

Buying Look for firm, smooth beets with fresh-looking tops; small, young beets are more tender and will cook faster than mature beets.

Storing Cut off the green tops to within 1 inch (2.5 cm) of the root, and refrigerate in a plastic bag for up to 2 weeks.

Quick tip Some stores carry precooked, packaged beets. You can also cook beets in advance and store them in an airtight container in the refrigerator for up to 3 days.

Using Add cooked, sliced beets to salads, or thinly slice raw golden beets and serve with a dip.

BELL PEPPERS

Buying Look for firm peppers with taut skin free of wrinkles or cracks. Buy organic when possible, as conventional bell peppers tend to have high levels of pesticides.

Storing Refrigerate in a paper bag in the crisper for up to 5 days.

Healthy tip The color and nutrient content of bell peppers change depending on how ripe they are; red, yellow, and orange bell peppers are much more nutritious than green.

Using Add sliced bell pepper to salads, stir-fries, or vegetable platters; roast red bell peppers whole (page 214), then peel and slice them and use in salads, pastas, sandwiches, and dips.

BERRIES
Includes blackberries, blueberries, cranberries, raspberries, strawberries

Buying Look for berries that are shiny, bright, and plump. Check the bottom of the container for moldy fruit. Buy organic berries when possible, as conventional ones tend to have high levels of pesticides.

Storing Refrigerate berries in a paper bag, or place in single layers between paper towels in an airtight container, for up to 2 days. Avoid washing berries until just before use, as the excess moisture can encourage mold growth.

Quick tip Nothing compares to fresh, seasonal berries. But when they're out of season, you can still get them in your diet by buying frozen or dried.

Using Sprinkle fresh or dried berries over low-fat or nonfat yogurt or cereal; add fresh or frozen berries to smoothies and desserts.

BROCCOLI
Includes broccoli, broccolini, broccoli rabe, Chinese broccoli

Buying Choose broccoli with tightly closed and uniformly green florets. Broccoli rabe should have crisp, bright green leaves and flowers that are just beginning to open.

Storing Refrigerate in a plastic bag in the crisper for up to 4 days (wrap broccoli rabe in a wet paper towel).

Quick tip Buy precut fresh or frozen florets, or cut up a head of broccoli and store until ready to use.

Using Cooked broccoli, whether steamed or roasted, makes a great side dish. It can also be eaten raw with a dip, or added to soups and stir-fries. Sautéed broccoli rabe is a nice addition to pastas and pizzas.

CABBAGE
Includes green and red cabbage, napa cabbage, Brussels sprouts, bok choy

Buying Cabbage heads should be firm and crisp; Brussels sprouts should be hard and bright green; bok choy should be crisp and firm, and not wilted.

Storing Refrigerate cabbage and Brussels sprouts in a plastic bag in the crisper for up to 1 week; bok choy will wilt within a few days.

Quick tip To save time, buy pre-shredded cabbage for slaws and salads, or shred a head of cabbage and store until ready to use.

Using Add shaved cabbage to salads and slaws; roast or sauté Brussels sprouts; add bok choy to stir-fries, soups, and noodle dishes.

CARROTS

Buying Choose firm, brightly colored carrots without splits or cracks.

Storing Refrigerate in a plastic bag in the crisper for up to 2 weeks (trim leafy green tops).

Prep tip You're more likely to snack on carrots during the week if you wash and cut them into matchsticks right after you buy them.

Using Add shredded carrots to salads, slaws, wraps, or muffin batter; eat raw carrots with hummus or low-fat yogurt dip.

CHERRIES

Buying Look for firm, shiny cherries with green stems. Avoid soft fruit with brown or moldy spots.

Storing Refrigerate in a plastic bag for up to 3 days, or freeze in a zippered plastic bag for up to 1 month.

Healthy tip Try to seek out sour cherries, which are very seasonal but widely available dried; they contain more nutrients than sweet cherries.

Using Eat fresh cherries on their own or with nonfat vanilla yogurt; add dried cherries to salads or trail mix, or use in baked goods.

CITRUS FRUITS

Includes oranges, tangerines, kumquats, grapefruits, lemons, limes

Buying Choose firm and blemish-free fruit that's heavy for its size and yields to gentle pressure. Opt for organic citrus fruits if you plan to use the zest.

Storing Refrigerate in a plastic bag for up to 3 weeks, or store in a single layer at cool room temperature for up to 1 week (citrus fruits can rot if crowded together).

Quick tip If you have some leftover citrus juice, pour it into ice-cube trays and freeze for later use.

Using Add citrus-fruit slices to salads; use the zest to brighten the flavors of many dishes; use the juice in drinks, dressings, and marinades.

CUCUMBERS

Buying Choose blemish-free cucumbers that are firm all the way to the tip. Hothouse cucumbers tend to be crunchier and more flavorful than common slicing cucumbers.

Storing Refrigerate in a plastic bag in the crisper for up to 1 week.

Prep tip To seed a cucumber, slice it in half lengthwise and use the tip of a spoon to scrape out the seeds.

Using Slice, dice, or grate and use in salads, sandwiches, and wraps.

DARK CHOCOLATE

Buying Choose high-quality bittersweet or semisweet dark chocolate that contains at least 60 percent cocoa. The lower the percentage of cocoa, the sweeter the chocolate will be.

Storing Wrap in plastic wrap or foil and store in a cool, dry place away from light and odors for up to 1 year. Never store dark chocolate in the refrigerator or freezer.

Healthy tip Milk chocolate and white chocolate contain much more sugar and milk solids than dark chocolate.

Using Savor a few squares of high-quality chocolate as a special treat; use in baked goods and puddings.

FENNEL

Buying Look for large, firm, pale green bulbs with bright green fronds.

Storing Refrigerate in a plastic bag in the crisper for up to 5 days.

Prep tip When slicing a fennel bulb, first remove the stalks and fronds, then slice the bulb in half vertically and remove the hard core.

Using Slice and add to salads; grill or braise and serve as a side dish.

GREEN BEANS

Buying Look for firm, bright green beans that snap when broken.

Storing Refrigerate in a plastic bag in the crisper for up to 1 week, or freeze for up to 3 months.

Quick tip If you can't find good-quality fresh green beans, all-natural frozen beans are a fine stand-in.

Using Steam, blanch, or sauté and serve as a side or in salads; serve fresh green beans with dips.

LEAFY GREENS

Includes arugula, chard, kale, romaine, spinach, watercress

Buying Look for crisp, deeply colored leaves without blemishes or a slimy coating. Buy organic when possible, as conventional greens tend to have high levels of pesticides.

Storing Store in a plastic bag in the crisper for 2–5 days. Wrap leaves in paper towels to keep extra crisp.

Prep tip Rinse greens well, being sure to remove all dirt and grit. If you are washing greens before storing them, remember to spin them dry; water can lead to spoilage.

Using Serve raw in salads; add chard, kale, or spinach to pastas and soups, or sauté and serve as a side dish.

MELONS

Includes cantaloupes, honeydews, seedless watermelons

Buying Look for hard melons that are heavy for their size; the blossom end should yield to gentle pressure and have a sweet aroma.

Storing Let whole melons ripen at room temperature; once ripe, refrigerate for up to 5 days.

Quick tip Slice a ripe melon and refrigerate the slices in an airtight container for up to 3 days.

Using Eat sliced melon as a snack; cube and add to salads; purée and add to beverages, or use in frozen treats.

MUSHROOMS

Buying Look for firm, smooth, and spongy mushrooms that aren't wet, slippery, or shriveled.

Storing Refrigerate in a paper bag for up to 3 days.

Prep tip Mushrooms absorb water easily; remove dirt with a damp cloth or paper towel, or rinse quickly under cold running water.

Using Slice and serve raw in salads; add to soups, stir-fries, and pastas; roast, grill, or sauté thick portobello mushrooms and add to sandwiches, or serve as a side dish.

NUTS

Includes almonds, cashews, peanuts, pecans, pistachios, walnuts

Buying Buy packaged nuts, or buy in bulk from a store that has a good product turnover. Experiment with different types of all-natural nut butters beyond peanut butter, including almond, walnut, and cashew butter.

Storing Some nuts are more perishable than others, but as a general rule, store nuts in an airtight container in a cool, dry place for up to 6 months, or in the refrigerator for up to 1 year.

Prep tip Don't skip the step of toasting nuts. It brings out their oils and flavors and usually takes less than 10 minutes.

Using Eat a few nuts as a snack out of hand; chop and add to granola, trail mix, salads, or baked goods; spread nut butter on bread or crackers, or eat with fruit or vegetables.

PEARS

Buying Look for firm fruit with smooth skin free of bruises and blemishes. Pears are ripe when the flesh near the stem end yields slightly to gentle pressure.

Storing Let ripen at room temperature in a paper bag; once ripe, refrigerate for up to 3 days.

Prep tip The flesh of cut pears browns quickly when exposed to air. To prevent this darkening, coat pieces evenly with a small amount of lemon juice.

Using Enjoy pears on their own; eat with nonfat or low-fat yogurt or cottage cheese; add to salads; use in baked dishes like crisps.

PEAS
Includes English peas, snow peas, sugar snap peas

Buying Choose firm, crisp peas with bright green pods.

Storing Refrigerate in a plastic bag in the crisper for up to 3 days.

Quick tip If you can't find good-quality fresh shelling peas, all-natural frozen peas are a fine stand-in.

Using Blanch or sauté fresh or frozen shelled English peas for a simple side dish; add sugar snap or snow peas to stir-fries and salads, or serve raw on vegetable platters.

POMEGRANATES
Buying Choose firm pomegranates that are heavy for their size; avoid bruised or shriveled fruits.

Storing If needed, let ripen at room temperature for 2–3 weeks; refrigerate ripe pomegranates for up to 1 month. Pomegranate seeds can be frozen for up to 3 months.

Quick tip To save time, look for packaged pomegranate seeds in the refrigerated produce section.

Using Add pomegranate seeds to salads and dips; use the juice in smoothies or frozen treats.

SEEDS
Includes flaxseed, pumpkin seeds, sesame seeds, sunflower seeds

Buying Buy packaged seeds, or buy in bulk from a store that has a good product turnover. If possible, smell seeds before buying them to make sure they don't have a rancid aroma.

Storing Refrigerate in an airtight container for up to 6 months, or freeze for up to 1 year.

Prep tip The next time you carve a pumpkin for Halloween, reserve the seeds for a healthy snack: Rinse and pat dry, sprinkle with salt, and toast in a dry frying pan over medium heat, stirring often, until the seeds are golden, 3–5 minutes.

Using Eat out of hand as a snack, add to trail mixes, or sprinkle over salads or soups.

SOYBEANS
Includes edamame, tofu

Buying If buying fresh edamame, look for bright green, plump pods. Choose organic, non-genetically modified beans when possible. Buy firm or extra-firm tofu for cooking.

Storing Refrigerate fresh edamame for up to 3 days; frozen will keep for a few months. Uncooked tofu will not keep long in the refrigerator.

Quick tip Precooked, marinated tofu is widely available, and can be eaten cold in salads and sandwiches.

Using Eat edamame as a snack, shelling as you go, or add to salads and dips. Use tofu in stir-fries and curries, or cook and add to salads and sandwiches.

STONE FRUITS
Includes apricots, peaches, plums

Buying Look for firm fruits that yield to gentle pressure. Buy organic peaches and nectarines when possible, as conventional ones tend to have high levels of pesticides.

Storing Let stone fruits ripen at room temperature; once ripe, refrigerate for up to 3 days.

Prep tip If stone fruits have been in the refrigerator, let them come to room temperature before eating: they will be sweeter and juicier.

Using Eat out of hand as a snack; slice and add to salads, salsas, or smoothies; grill and serve as an appetizer or dessert.

SWEET POTATOES
Buying Choose firm orange-fleshed sweet potatoes (often labeled as yams) that are free of cracks, bruises, or soft spots.

Storing Store in a cool, dry place for up to 2 weeks; do not refrigerate.

Quick tip If you're short on time, remember that sliced or cubed sweet potatoes will cook much faster than whole ones.

Using Roast, steam, or boil and serve as a side dish; cut into matchsticks and bake to make oven fries.

TOMATOES
Buying Look for firm, plump tomatoes that yield to gentle pressure. Vine-ripened tomatoes, available during the summer months, will have the best flavor. Choose from an array of colorful heirloom tomatoes when available at the market.

Storing Let ripen at room temperature; do not refrigerate.

Quick tip Have a good supply of low-sodium, all-natural canned tomatoes on hand for adding to pastas and soups when tomatoes are out of season.

Using Slice or chop and eat raw in salads, sandwiches, and salsas; add to soups, pastas, and sauces.

TROPICAL FRUITS
Includes kiwifruits, mangoes, papayas, pineapples

Buying Look for soft fruits that yield to gentle pressure but aren't squishy or shriveled. Ripe pineapples will be slightly soft to the touch, and the stem end should have a sweet aroma.

Storing Let ripen at room temperature; refrigerate cut fruit in an airtight container for up to 3 days.

Quick tip For a quick snack that requires little prep work, halve a ripe kiwifruit lengthwise and scoop out the flesh with a spoon.

Using Slice and eat as a snack; add to salads, salsas, and smoothies.

WHOLE GRAINS
Includes brown rice, buckwheat, corn, oats, quinoa, rye, whole wheat

Buying Buy minimally processed grains in bulk from a store that has a good product turnover. Look for breads, crackers, tortillas, cereals, and other dry goods made with whole grains rather than processed.

Storing Store dry goods such as flour and whole grains in a cool, dry place for 2–6 months, depending on the grain, or store in the refrigerator for longer. Eat bread and tortillas within a few days, or by the expiration date listed on the package (or wrap tightly and freeze for longer).

Prep tip Prepare a batch of brown rice, quinoa, or oatmeal on the weekend and refrigerate it for meals on-the-go during the week.

Using Flavor cooked grains like quinoa and brown rice with olive oil and fresh herbs and serve as a side dish; eat oatmeal for breakfast or use in baking; use buckwheat and whole-wheat flour for making pancakes and baked goods.

WINTER SQUASH

Includes acorn, butternut, delicata, kabocha, pumpkin

Buying Look for firm squash that does not yield to pressure and is free of soft spots or bruises.

Storing Store at cool room temperature for 1–6 months, depending on the variety.

Quick tip To save time, purchase precubed squash or even all-natural, 100 percent canned pumpkin purée.

Using Roast or steam squash wedges and serve as a side dish, or add cubed squash to soups; use canned pumpkin purée for baking.

If you let superfoods play a starring role in your meals, these ingredients will make a great supporting cast. Enjoy lean proteins, eggs, dairy, heart–healthy oils, and sweeteners in moderation. Use a heavy hand with herbs, spices, and other flavor boosters.

OTHER HEALTHY INGREDIENTS

HEART-HEALTHY OILS

Choose your oil wisely to keep your meals at their nutritional best. The following five types are especially good choices.

canola Light in color and bland, choose canola oil for all your general cooking and baking needs.

grapeseed Like canola oil, grapeseed oil is a good all-purpose choice when you need a flavorless oil. It's especially good for high-temperature cooking.

olive Extra-virgin olive oil has a fruity, slightly peppery flavor and can be used uncooked in dressings or lightly cooked for sautéing.

peanut With its hint of nuttiness and high smoke point, peanut oil can be used for salads or cooking.

sesame The lighter colored, more refined sesame oil can be used for light sautéing, but the darker, more aromatic oil is best reserved sparingly as a seasoning.

SEAFOOD

Quick-cooking seafood provides a low-fat source of protein to round out your meals. Healthful fish choices include wild-caught Alaskan salmon (or wild canned salmon), albacore tuna, and a variety of white fish, such as domestically farmed tilapia and Alaskan halibut. Sensible shellfish picks include wild shrimp, scallops, and squid.

When buying fresh fish and shellfish, look for a moist, bright appearance and fresh, clean scent. Store fish in the coldest part of the refrigerator for up to 2 days, or tightly wrapped in the freezer for up to 1 month. Store shellfish in the refrigerator until ready to serve, up to 1 day. To be sure you are making the best seafood choices for cooking, visit montereybayaquarium.org and click on the Seafood Watch link.

POULTRY & MEAT

Rich in protein, poultry and meat can be great additions to a busy, healthful lifestyle if you choose lean, fast-cooking cuts. Both skinless chicken and turkey breasts are ideal for quick dinners, as they are low in fat and cook up in minutes. Similarly, pork tenderloin can lend variety to your weekly meals. Beef, too, can be a sensible choice if you eat it in moderation. Flank and skirt steak are quick-cooking and versatile options. Some authorities claim that organic, grass-fed beef boasts increased nutritional value over traditional corn-fed beef, and it's becoming more widely available.

Purchase poultry and meat from a local butcher with a reputation for quality and a high turnover. Store both in the coldest part of the refrigerator and use as soon as possible, or by the sell-by date on the packaging.

EGGS & DAIRY

Packed with protein and calcium, low-fat and nonfat dairy products are a boon to a healthy lifestyle. Eggs are one of the best quick-cooking ingredients for healthful meals, while yogurt is a versatile staple that no healthy-minded eater should do without. Look for cheeses that are made with part-skim milk to add creaminess to dishes without a lot of extra fat, and use small amounts of flavorful cheese as an occasional high-fat indulgence.

For the most delicious and vibrantly colored eggs, a farmers' market is your best source. For everyday shopping, look for organic, cage-free large eggs. Purchase yogurt and cheese from a store with high turnover. Store eggs and dairy in the refrigerator and use by the sell-by date on the packaging.

FRESH HERBS
Replete with healthful properties, popular cooking herbs include basil, cilantro, mint, oregano, parsley, rosemary, sage, and thyme.

Choose fresh herbs that look bright, fragrant, and healthy. Avoid those that have silted, yellowed, or blackened leaves or moldy stems. Wrap fresh herbs in damp paper towels then store in a plastic bag in the refrigerator for 3–5 days.

SPICES
Popular spices with nutritional benefits include cinnamon, cumin, curry powder, nutmeg, paprika, and turmeric.

For the best flavor, buy your spices whole and grind them in a spice grinder just before use. Purchase spices in the smallest amounts you can, as they lose flavor over time. Store in tightly closed containers in a cool, dark cupboard. Whole spices will keep for up to 1 year; ground spices should be used within 6 months.

VINEGAR
A good way to boost flavor without adding calories, vinegar is an essential pantry staple. Types of vinegar include balsamic, cider, red and white wine, and rice wine.

Most vinegars can be stored indefinitely in a cool, dark place.

AROMATICS
There are a handful of ingredients considered "aromatics," which add a lot more than just aroma to a dish. Chiles, garlic, ginger, onions, and shallots all possess their own unique healthful qualities that pump up the nutritional value of a dish at the same time as they deliver flavor.

As with other vegetables, choose aromatics that seem fresh, firm, and heavy for their size from a quality source with high turnover. Store fresh chiles as you would bell peppers (see page 15). Garlic, onions, and shallots should be stored in a cool, dark place, while green onions can be refrigerated for up to 1 week. Store fresh ginger in the refrigerator for up to 3 weeks, grating or cutting off slices as needed.

NATURAL SWEETENERS
Look beyond refined white sugar to these minimally processed sweeteners that contain beneficial health properties.

agave This super-sweet plant nectar, an all-natural substitute for processed sugar, is now widely available in most food stores.

honey Choose all-natural, raw honey for the highest nutritional value. Store in an airtight container in a cool, dry place.

maple syrup Choose pure maple syrup, preferably USDA Grade B. Refrigerate once opened.

A balanced breakfast sets the stage for a day of healthy eating, providing you with the energy you need to make it through your busy morning.

BREAKFAST

QUICK-FIX IDEAS FOR BREAKFAST

EAT IT ON THE RUN

FRUIT SMOOTHIE Chill an insulated beverage container in the freezer while you make the Blueberry-Pomegranate Smoothie (page 29) or Rise and Shine Smoothie (page 30), or make your own—using fresh or frozen fruit, nonfat or low-fat yogurt, and fruit juice. Pour the smoothie in the cold container and close tightly. Rinse out the blender before you leave, to ease cleanup later.

BREAKFAST PITA Stuff your favorite egg scramble into a warmed whole-wheat pita pocket. Add a superfood such as chopped tomato, baby spinach leaves, or cubed avocado. Wrap in foil or plastic wrap and eat out of hand.

NUT BUTTER–FRUIT WRAP Spread peanut, almond, or cashew butter on a whole-wheat tortilla. Top with apple slices or dried cherries or cranberries, pressing them gently into the nut butter to help them adhere. Add a drizzle of honey, if you like. Fold in two sides of the tortilla and then roll it up like a burrito; wrap in foil or plastic wrap and eat out of hand.

PACK IT TO GO

OATMEAL Prepare your favorite hot breakfast cereal, such as Apple-Cinnamon Oatmeal (page 35) or Whole-Wheat Farina (page 37). Meanwhile, fill an insulated beverage container with hot water to warm it. When the cereal is ready, pour out the water and add the cereal to the container. Add any desired toppings, like nonfat or low-fat milk, dark agave nectar or maple syrup, ground cinnamon, chopped walnuts, or fresh or dried fruit.

BREAKFAST BOWL Fill a to-go container with a medley of your favorite breakfast ingredients. Try a chopped hard-boiled egg, cubed avocado, and cucumber slices sprinkled with sea salt and lime; low-fat cottage cheese topped with tomato slices and fresh herbs, or pear slices and ground cinnamon; or plain low-fat or nonfat yogurt topped with fruit and a sprinkle of the Crunchy Breakfast Topping (right).

MAKE IT AHEAD

CRUNCHY BREAKFAST TOPPING Combine equal parts raw sunflower and sesame seeds in a small frying pan and toast over medium heat until fragrant and lightly colored, about 3 minutes. Pour into a jar or airtight container and add equal parts toasted wheat germ, ground flaxseed, and brown sugar. Cover and shake to combine. Store, tightly covered, in the refrigerator for up to 3 months. To serve, sprinkle the mixture over low-fat or nonfat yogurt or sliced fresh fruit such as mangoes, berries, or plums.

FRITTATA WEDGES Prepare the Frittata with Turkey Sausage and Arugula (page 48), or create your own frittata using a combination of chopped vegetables, cooked lean meats, and/or cheeses. Cool and cut into wedges. Wrap the wedges in foil, place in a zippered plastic bag, and store in the freezer for up to 3 months. To serve, unwrap and cook in the microwave on high power for 30–45 seconds.

GRANOLA OR MUESLI Make a big batch of Maple–Almond Granola (page 33) or muesli (page 38) on the weekend and store in a jar or airtight container for up to 2 weeks. Eat with nonfat or low-fat yogurt, kefir, or milk.

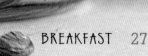

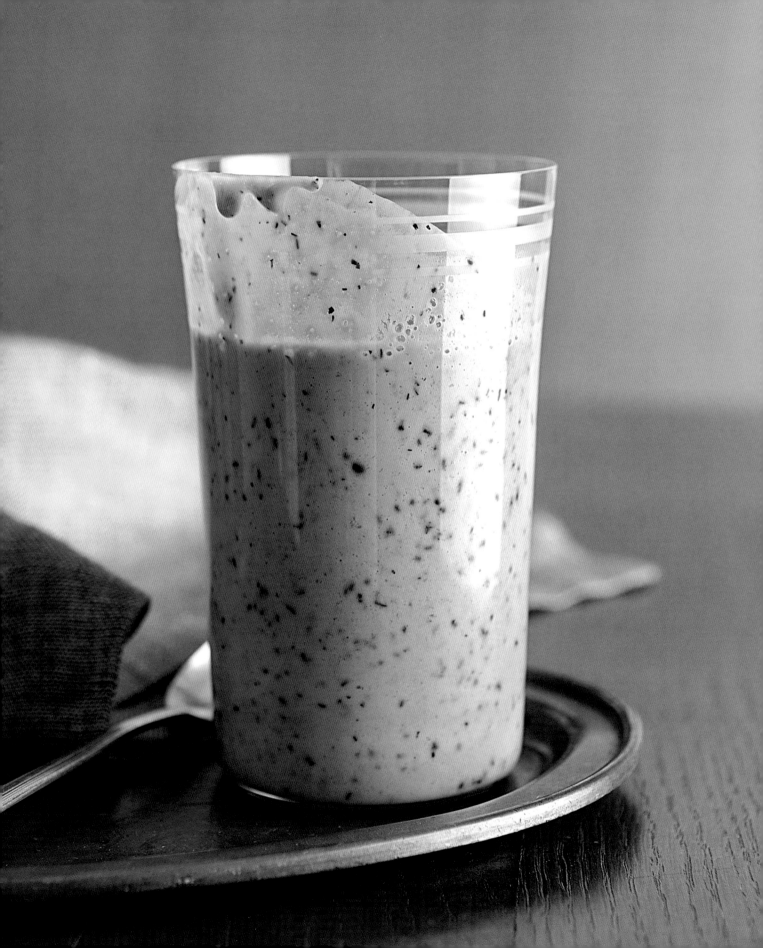

If you have fresh blueberries on hand, by all means use them, but add a few ice cubes before blending to chill the smoothie. Keep an insulated beverage container stashed in the freezer—it will come in handy if you like to take your smoothies to go.

BLUEBERRY-POMEGRANATE SMOOTHIE

ripe banana, 1

frozen blueberries, ½ cup (2 oz/60 g)

honey, 1 Tbsp

pomegranate juice, ½ cup (4 fl oz/125 ml)

plain nonfat yogurt, 1 cup (8 oz/250 g)

MAKES 2 SERVINGS

1 Peel banana and cut into chunks.

2 In a blender or food processor, combine banana, blueberries, honey, and pomegranate juice and process to a coarse purée, 30–45 seconds. Add yogurt and whirl until smooth.

3 Pour into glasses and serve right away, or transfer to insulated beverage containers and take to go.

What could be better than a healthy breakfast that comes together in less than a minute? Each of the 5 ingredients here packs a nutritional wallop.

bananas
- Excellent source of vitamin B6
- Good source of both potassium and fiber
- Help maintain good blood pressure and digestive health

pomegranate juice
- Rich in antioxidants
- Good source of folate and potassium
- Linked to heart health and cancer prevention

per serving 220 calories, 8 g protein, 47 g carbs, .5 g fat (0 g saturated fat), 0 mg cholesterol, 3 g fiber, 100 mg sodium

The bright flavors of citrus, mango, and ginger shine in this sunny orange smoothie. If you're short on time, don't worry about peeling the fresh ginger root: just rinse it well and run it crosswise through a fine grater.

RISE & SHINE SMOOTHIE

With two tasty, gut-friendly ingredients and a blend of tart citrus juice and spicy ginger, this will get your body and mind going before a busy day.

mangoes
- Packed with fiber
- Good source of vitamin E and beta-carotene, antioxidants that support eye health
- Excellent source of vitamins A and C

nonfat yogurt
- Excellent source of calcium
- Contains beneficial bacteria that aids digestion
- Look for "live active cultures" on the label

per serving 190 calories, 5 g protein, 44 g carbs, .5 g fat (0 g saturated fat), 0 mg cholesterol, 2 g fiber, 35 mg sodium

ripe mango, 1
fresh orange juice, ¾–1 cup (6–8 fl oz/180–250 ml)
vanilla nonfat yogurt, ½ cup (4 oz/125 g)
fresh ginger, ½ tsp grated
honey, 1 Tbsp
fresh lime juice, 1 Tbsp
MAKES 2 SERVINGS

1 Hold mango upright on a cutting board. Using a sharp chef's knife, make downward cuts along each flat side of pit to separate from flesh. Remove skin with a vegetable peeler and cut flesh into chunks.

2 In a blender, whirl mango, ¾ cup (6 fl oz/180 ml) orange juice, yogurt, ginger, honey, and lime juice until smooth. Add up to ¼ cup (2 fl oz/60 ml) more orange juice as needed for desired consistency.

3 Pour into glasses and serve right away, or transfer to insulated beverage containers and take to go.

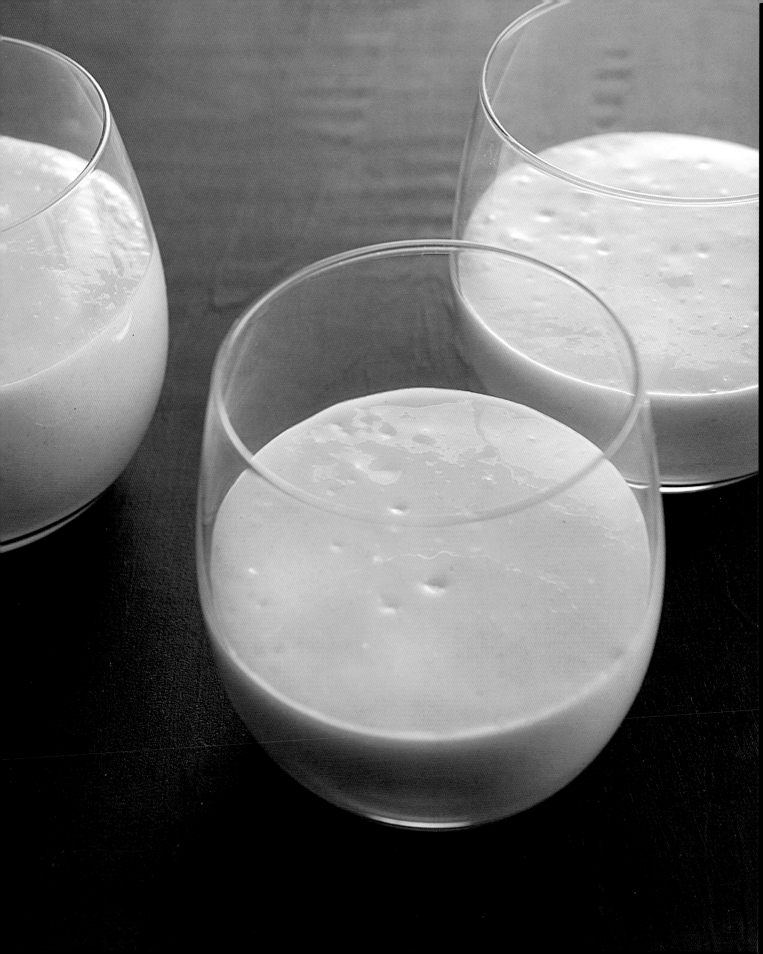

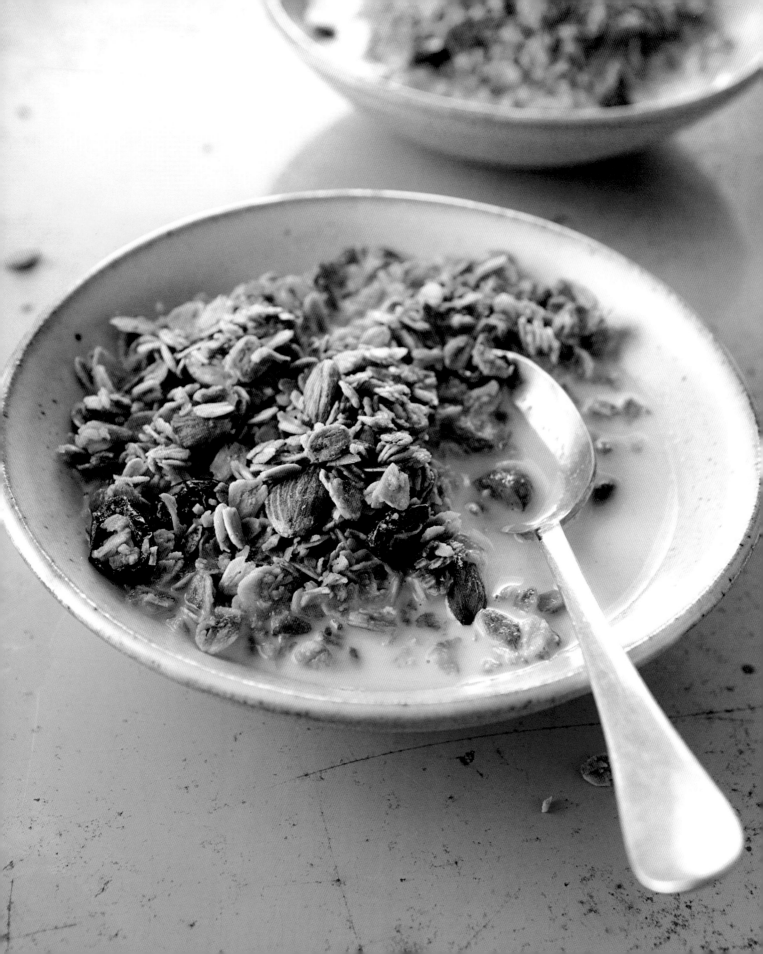

Lightly sweetened with honey and maple syrup, this crunchy fruit-and-nut granola will become a staple in your home. Make a big batch and keep it on hand to sprinkle over low-fat or nonfat milk or yogurt for an easy, wholesome start to the day.

MAPLE-ALMOND GRANOLA

canola oil, 2 tsp plus ¼ cup
(2 fl oz/60 ml)

pure grade-B maple syrup, ½ cup
(5½ oz/170 g)

honey, ¼ cup (3 oz/90 g)

salt, ¼ tsp

rolled oats, 4 cups (12 oz/375 g)

almonds, 1¼ cups (5 oz/155 g),
coarsely chopped

dried cranberries or currants, ¼ cup
(1 oz/30 g)

MAKES 12 SERVINGS

1 Preheat oven to 325°F (165°C). Lightly grease a 12-by-15-inch (30-by-38-cm) baking pan with 2 teaspoons oil.

2 In a large bowl, whisk together ¼ cup oil, maple syrup, honey, and salt. Stir in oats and almonds, mixing to coat them completely. Spread evenly in prepared pan and bake, stirring every 10 minutes, until mixture is golden brown, 30–35 minutes.

3 Let cool completely, then stir in cranberries. Store granola in an airtight container at room temperature for up to 2 weeks.

Purchased cereal can be high in fat and sugar, but if you make it yourself with a heart-healthy oil, granola can be a sensible addition to any eating plan.

oats
- Rich in beta-glucan, shown to lower cholesterol
- Excellent source of zinc, iron, and magnesium
- Source of antioxidants linked to cardiovascular health

canola oil
- Excellent source of heart-smart omega-3 fatty acids
- Rich in monounsaturated fats
- Flavorless, so it's a good choice in sweet recipes

per serving 400 calories,
12 g protein, 55 g carbs,
16 g fat (1.5 g saturated fat),
0 mg cholesterol, 7 g fiber,
50 mg sodium

Bake a batch of these tender muffins anytime and freeze them so you can reheat them for weekday morning breakfasts. For a tropical variation, substitute unsweetened shredded coconut and diced dried pineapple for the walnuts and raisins.

CARROT MUFFINS

Replacing a portion of the all-purpose flour with whole-wheat flour adds nutrients and fiber and a pleasing nutty flavor.

carrots
- Deep yellow-orange pigment is linked to reduced risk of cardiovascular disease
- May help protect against colon cancer
- Excellent source of vitamin A

whole-wheat flour
- Rich in insoluble fiber linked to improved digestive health
- Provides antioxidants that enhance heart health
- Source of complex carbs, which help regulate blood sugar

per muffin 270 calories,
5 g protein, 32 g carbs,
14 g fat (1.5 g saturated fat),
40 mg cholesterol, 2 g fiber,
180 mg sodium

all-purpose flour, 1 cup (5 oz/155 g)
whole-wheat flour, ⅔ cup (3½ oz/105 g)
baking soda, ½ tsp
baking powder, ½ tsp
salt, ¼ tsp
large eggs, 2
vegetable oil, ½ cup (4 fl oz/125 ml)
light brown sugar, ½ cup firmly packed (3½ oz/105 g)

carrots, 3, peeled and grated (about 1½ cups/9 oz/280 g)
low-fat (1%) milk, ½ cup (4 fl oz/125 ml)
chopped walnuts, ¼ cup (1 oz/30 g)
golden raisins, ¼ cup (1½ oz/45 g)

MAKES 10 MUFFINS

1 Preheat oven to 375°F (190°C). Line 10 cups of a standard muffin pan with paper liners.

2 In a medium bowl, stir together flours, baking soda, baking powder, and salt.

3 In a large bowl, whisk together eggs, oil, and brown sugar. Stir in carrots. Add flour mixture and milk and stir just until dry ingredients are evenly moistened. Gently stir in walnuts and raisins.

4 Spoon batter into prepared cups, filling each about three-fourths full. Bake until tops of muffins are set and spring back when lightly pressed, 20–25 minutes. Let cool slightly, then lift muffins carefully from pan and transfer to a wire rack to cool completely. Store in an airtight container at room temperature for up to 2 days, or pack into zippered freezer bags and freeze for up to 1 month.

Maple sugar, available in many gourmet shops and well-stocked supermarkets, has a rich, mellow, concentrated sweetness. If you can't find it, maple syrup or dark brown cane sugar will do. For extra sweetness, sprinkle dried cranberries on top along with the walnuts.

APPLE-CINNAMON OATMEAL

chopped walnuts, ½ cup (2 oz/60 g)

rolled oats, 1 cup (3 oz/90 g)

dried apples, ½ cup (1½ oz/45 g), chopped

ground cinnamon, ¾ tsp

maple sugar, 2 Tbsp

MAKES 4 SERVINGS

1 Preheat oven to 350°F (180°C). Spread walnuts on a baking sheet and toast until lightly browned and fragrant, about 10 minutes. Immediately pour onto a plate to cool. Set aside.

2 In a saucepan, combine oats, apples, cinnamon, and 2 cups (16 fl oz/500 ml) water. Bring to a simmer over medium-high heat. Reduce heat to medium and cook, stirring occasionally, until water is absorbed and oats are creamy, 7–10 minutes.

3 Spoon oatmeal into bowls and top each serving with walnuts and maple sugar. Serve right away.

Here's a comforting and nutritious recipe that can be made entirely from healthful pantry staples.

apples
- Contain pectin, a soluble fiber shown to lower cholesterol
- Rich in quercetin, a compound that helps regulate blood sugar
- Look for dried apples with the peels for maximum nutrition

walnuts
- Contain more heart-healthy omega-3 fats than any other nut
- May protect against heart disease and dementia

per serving 290 calories, 9 g protein, 39 g carbs, 12 g fat (1.5 g saturated fat), 0 mg cholesterol, 6 g fiber, 10 mg sodium

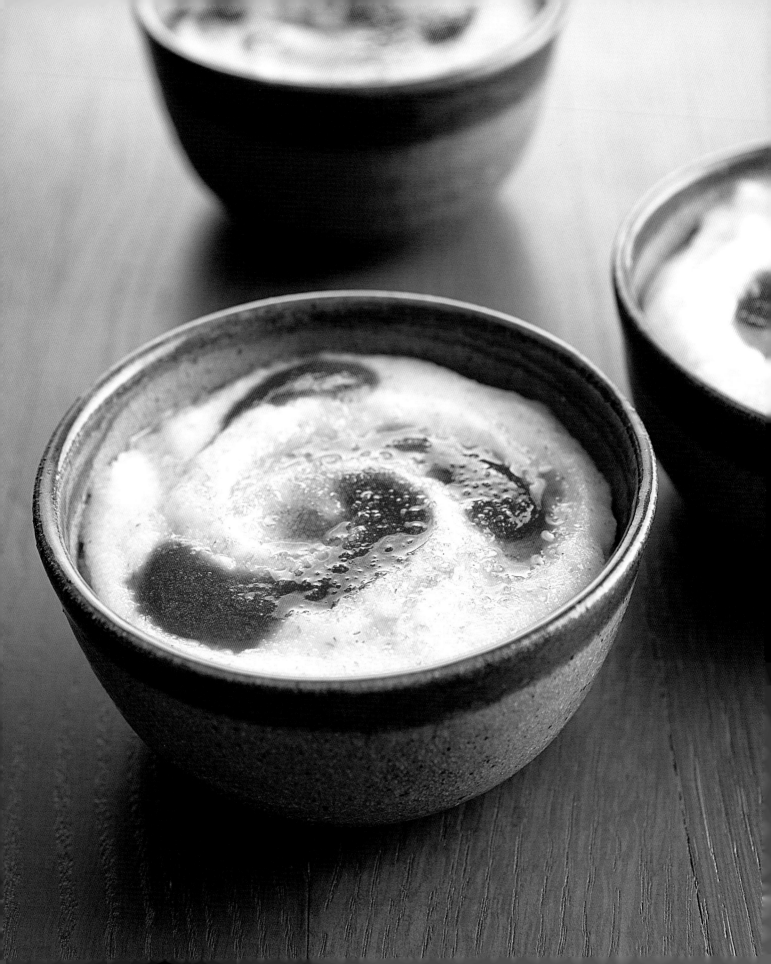

A bright berry sauce swirled into creamy whole-wheat cereal is a sublime alternative to oatmeal. Serve this comforting dish with a splash of milk and a sprinkle of turbinado sugar, if you like. If you don't have fresh berries, thawed frozen ones will do.

WHOLE-WHEAT FARINA WITH BERRY SWIRL

sea salt, a pinch

whole-wheat farina, 1 cup (6 oz/185 g)

fresh berries such as raspberries, blackberries, or blueberries, or a combination, 1 cup (4 oz/125 g)

sugar, 2 Tbsp

fresh lemon juice, ¼ tsp

MAKES 4 SERVINGS

1 In a saucepan, bring 3 cups (24 fl oz/750 ml) water to a boil over high heat. Stir in salt. Slowly whisk in farina and reduce heat to low. Cover and cook, stirring occasionally, until grains are tender, 4–6 minutes.

2 In a blender or food processor, whirl berries and sugar until smooth. Pour purée through a fine-mesh sieve into a small bowl, using a rubber spatula or wooden spoon to press on solids and extract as much juice as possible. Discard solids. Stir in lemon juice.

3 Spoon farina into 4 bowls, dividing it evenly. Top each with a swirl of berry purée. Serve right away.

For the most nutrition and best texture and flavor, choose stone-ground, organic farina over processed or instant cereal.

raspberries
- Contain a high concentration of ellagic acid, a cancer fighter
- Excellent source of vitamin C and manganese, which keep cells healthy by protecting them from free radical damage
- Especially rich in fiber

per serving 200 calories, 5 g protein, 44 g carbs, 0 g fat (0 g saturated fat), 0 mg cholesterol, 3 g fiber, 35 mg sodium

The now widely popular cereal called *muesli,* which originated in Switzerland, is by rough definition a mixture of rolled oats, dried fruit, and nuts. This version adds whole-grain heft with puffed brown rice and bran flakes. Pour it over milk or yogurt for a fiber-rich breakfast.

MUESLI WITH ALMONDS, COCONUT & DRIED FRUIT

A generous sprinkling of nuts, seeds, and dried fruits adds additional texture, fiber, and protein to a morning favorite.

sunflower seeds
- Packed with antioxidants like vitamin E and selenium
- Good source of minerals such as copper, potassium, and zinc
- Rich in compounds that help lower cholesterol

dried cherries
- Contain melatonin, linked to improved sleep
- May relieve muscle and joint soreness
- Source of antioxidants that help reduce inflammation

per serving 230 calories, 7 g protein, 31 g carbs, 10 g fat (2.5 g saturated fat), 0 mg cholesterol, 6 g fiber, 20 mg sodium

rolled oats, 2 cups (6 oz/185 g)

almonds, 1 cup (5 oz/155 g), chopped

unsweetened or lightly sweetened puffed brown rice cereal, 1 cup (2 oz/60 g)

unsweetened or lightly sweetened bran flakes, ½ cup (1¼ oz/37 g)

unsweetened flaked coconut, ⅓ cup (1½ oz/45 g)

toasted pumpkin seeds, 3 Tbsp

toasted sunflower seeds, 3 Tbsp

dried cherries or raisins, ¾ cup (about 4 oz/125 g)

pitted dates, ½ cup (3 oz/90 g) chopped

MAKES 15 SERVINGS

1 Preheat oven to 350°F (180°C).

2 Place oats and almonds on a baking sheet and toast in oven until fragrant and just starting to turn golden, about 10 minutes. Remove from oven and let cool completely.

3 Transfer oats and nuts to a large bowl. Add brown rice cereal, bran flakes, coconut, pumpkin seeds, sunflower seeds, cherries, and dates and stir to distribute ingredients evenly. Store in an airtight container at room temperature for up to 2 weeks.

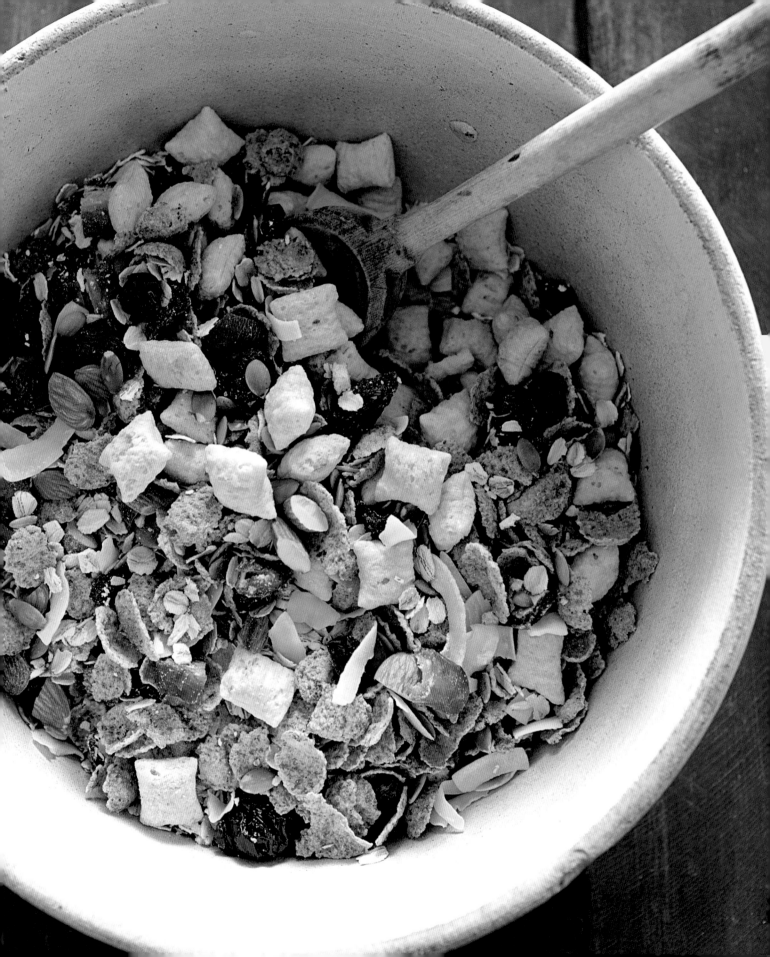

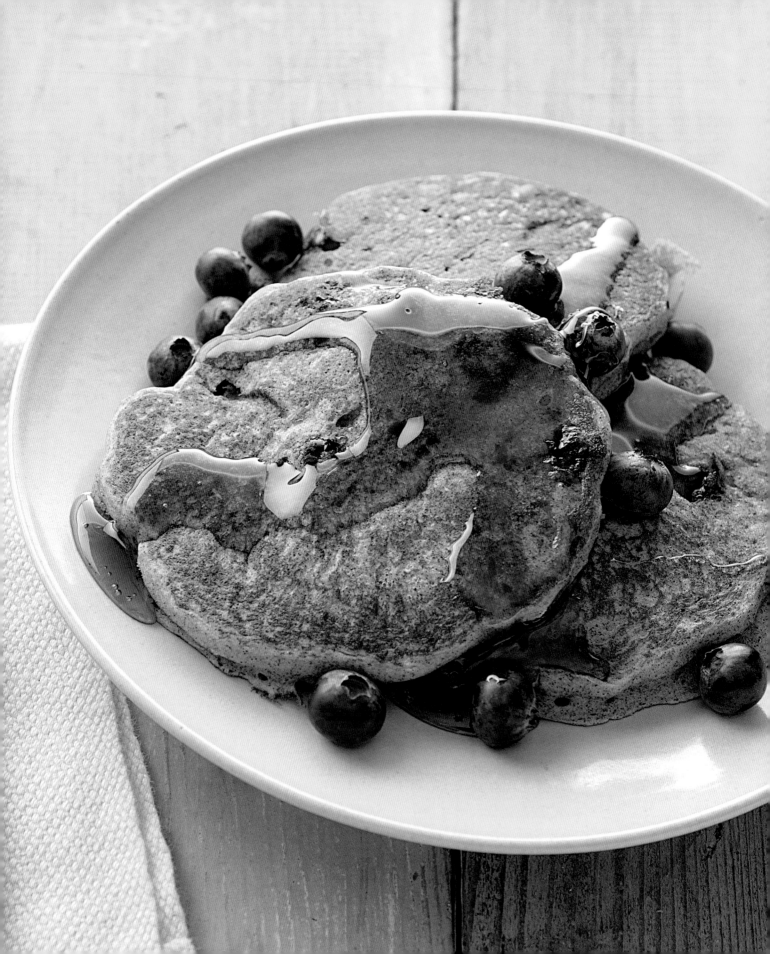

Tart-sweet blueberries give these tender pancakes bursts of fruit flavor; if you have extra fresh berries on hand, use them as a garnish. Freeze leftover pancakes in a zippered plastic bag, between sheets of waxed paper, for up to 1 month.

BUCKWHEAT-BLUEBERRY PANCAKES

all-purpose flour, 1¼ cups (6½ oz/200 g)

buckwheat flour, ¾ cup (4 oz/125 g)

baking powder, 1½ tsp

baking soda, 1½ tsp

salt, ¼ tsp

large eggs, 2

low-fat (1%) buttermilk, 2½ cups (20 fl oz/625 ml)

canola oil, 2 Tbsp plus 2 tsp

fresh or frozen blueberries, 1 cup (4 oz/125 g)

pure maple syrup, ½ cup (5½ oz/170 g), warmed

MAKES 6 SERVINGS

1 In a large bowl, stir together flours, baking powder, baking soda, and salt. In a small bowl, whisk together eggs, buttermilk, and 2 tablespoons oil until well blended. Stir egg mixture into flour mixture just until blended, then gently fold in blueberries.

2 Preheat oven to 200°F (95°C). Heat a 12-inch (30-cm) nonstick frying pan or a nonstick griddle over medium heat. Coat pan lightly with 2 teaspoons oil and carefully wipe out any excess with a paper towel. Pour batter into pan in about ⅓-cup (2½–fl oz/70-ml) portions and cook until pancakes are browned on the bottoms and bubbles form on top, about 2 minutes.

3 Flip pancakes and cook until second sides are browned, 1½–2 minutes longer. Transfer to a platter and keep warm in oven while you cook remaining pancakes. Serve warm with maple syrup.

Buckwheat flour lends flavor and whole-grain goodness to a classic pancake recipe. Using low-fat buttermilk keeps the fat content in check.

buckwheat flour
- Rich in magnesium, which promotes blood-vessel health
- Helps regulate blood sugar

blueberries
- Excellent source of antioxidants linked to improved memory
- Rich in flavonoids, which protect against cancer and guard heart health
- Low in calories and high in fiber

per serving 350 calories, 10 g protein, 57 g carbs, 9 g fat (1.5 g saturated fat), 65 mg cholesterol, 3 g fiber, 670 mg sodium

Pumpkin adds a rich, moist texture to these crisp, golden waffles. White whole-wheat flour is ground from a variety of wheat that has a lighter color and milder flavor than standard whole-wheat flour. If your market doesn't carry it, you can substitute regular whole-wheat.

PUMPKIN WAFFLES WITH ORANGE & CINNAMON

This recipe is a good one to serve during the fall months. Its comforting flavor is reminiscent of pumpkin pie, without all the saturated fat.

pumpkin

- Rich in carotenoids, which protect against heart disease and some cancers
- Packed with vitamin A and fiber
- Look for cans that contain 100 percent pumpkin

cinnamon

- Helps balance blood sugar
- Prevents formation of blood clots
- Its aroma enhances memory and mental function

per serving 420 calories,
11 g protein, 49 g carbs,
20 g fat (2.5 g saturated fat),
95 mg cholesterol, 4 g fiber,
580 mg sodium

all-purpose flour, 1 cup (5 oz/155 g)

white whole-wheat flour, ½ cup (2½ oz/75 g)

sugar, 2 Tbsp

baking powder, 1 Tbsp

ground cinnamon, ¾ tsp

salt, ¼ tsp

low-fat (1%) milk, 1 cup (8 fl oz/250 ml)

canned pumpkin purée, ½ cup (4 oz/125 g)

large eggs, 2

canola oil, ¼ cup (2 fl oz/60 ml) plus 2 tsp

pure vanilla extract, 1 tsp

finely grated orange zest, 1 Tbsp

MAKES 4 SERVINGS

1 In a small bowl, stir together flours, sugar, baking powder, cinnamon, and salt. In a large bowl, whisk together milk, pumpkin, eggs, ¼ cup oil, vanilla, and orange zest. Add flour mixture and stir just until combined.

2 Preheat oven to 200°F (95°C). Brush waffle iron lightly with 2 teaspoons oil, wiping off any excess with a paper towel. Preheat to medium per manufacturer's instructions. Spoon about ½ cup (4 fl oz/125 ml) batter onto hot waffle iron, spreading it out to the edges. Cook until golden brown, 3–5 minutes. Open iron carefully and transfer waffle to a plate. Keep warm in oven while you repeat to make 3 more waffles. Serve right away.

These satisfying breakfast potatoes are delicious alongside any egg dish, or even a tofu scramble (page 44). Use the roasting time to prepare the rest of your breakfast components. Use a combination of sweet potatoes and garnet yams for a pretty orange-and-red dish.

ROASTED SWEET POTATO HASH

orange-fleshed sweet potatoes, 2 lb (1 kg), peeled and cut into ½-inch (12-mm) cubes

shallots, 8 oz (250 g), halved, or quartered if large

garlic cloves, 6, smashed

olive oil, 2 Tbsp

coarse sea salt, ½ tsp

freshly ground pepper, to taste

fresh thyme, 1 tsp chopped

MAKES 4 SERVINGS

1 Preheat oven to 400°F (200°C).

2 Put sweet potatoes, shallots, and garlic in a roasting pan. Drizzle with olive oil and sprinkle with salt and pepper. Toss to mix well and coat potatoes thoroughly with oil and seasonings.

3 Roast, stirring every 10 minutes to help with even browning, until potatoes are tender, 25–30 minutes. Stir in thyme and serve right away.

Here, sweet potatoes stand in for white potatoes in a flavorful, colorful, and nutrient-dense version of a classic brunch dish.

sweet potatoes
- Outstanding source of vitamin A, beta-carotene, and vitamin C
- Provide plenty of potassium and fiber
- Help regulate blood sugar

fresh thyme
- Rich in vitamin K, needed for blood clotting and bone health
- Contains a wide variety of flavonoids, which act as antioxidants

per serving 300 calories, 5 g protein, 57 g carbs, 7 g fat (1 g saturated fat), 0 mg cholesterol, 7 g fiber, 380 mg sodium

This hearty breakfast dish cooks up quickly and is a delicious alternative to the usual egg scramble. Sweet corn adds color and crunch (frozen will do just as well as summer fresh), while fresh ginger, curry powder, and cilantro provide a boost of flavor.

TOFU SCRAMBLE WITH CORN, MUSHROOMS & BELL PEPPERS

Curry powder is a blend of potent spices, including cumin, turmeric, and chiles. Its unique flavor helps take good-for-you tofu to new heights.

tofu
- Provides complete vegetarian protein
- Linked to heart health
- Contains the omega-3 fat alpha linolenic acid

curry powder
- Contains cumin to aid digestion
- Rich in turmeric, a natural cancer fighter
- Chiles provide capsaicin, which boosts metabolism

per serving 230 calories, 13 g protein, 17 g carbs, 14 g fat (2.5 g saturated fat), 0 mg cholesterol, 3 g fiber, 200 mg sodium

olive oil, 2 tsp plus 2 Tbsp

fresh lime juice, 2 Tbsp

low-sodium soy sauce, 4 tsp

sweet curry powder, 1 Tbsp

fresh ginger, 1-inch (2.5-cm) piece, peeled and grated or minced

firm tofu, 1 lb (500 g), drained and cut into 1-inch (2.5-cm) cubes

cremini mushrooms, 8 oz (250 g), sliced

garlic, 2 cloves, pressed or minced

green onions, 1 bunch, white and pale green parts, thinly sliced

red bell pepper, 1, seeded and thinly sliced

sweet yellow corn kernels, 1 cup (6 oz/185 g), thawed frozen or cut from about 2 ears of corn

fresh cilantro, 2 Tbsp chopped

MAKES 4 SERVINGS

1 In a large bowl, stir together 2 teaspoons olive oil, lime juice, soy sauce, curry powder, and ginger. Add tofu and stir gently to coat.

2 Heat 2 tablespoons olive oil in a large frying pan over medium-high heat. Add mushrooms and cook, stirring often, until they release their juices and begin to brown, 3–4 minutes. Stir in garlic and green onions and cook until garlic is fragrant and onions are softened, about 1 minute. Stir in bell pepper and corn and cook until softened, 1–2 minutes.

3 Add tofu with its marinade. Stir to combine and break up pieces of tofu slightly. Cook, stirring often, until liquid is evaporated and parts of mixture are crusty and browned, about 5 minutes longer. Remove from heat, stir in cilantro, and serve right away.

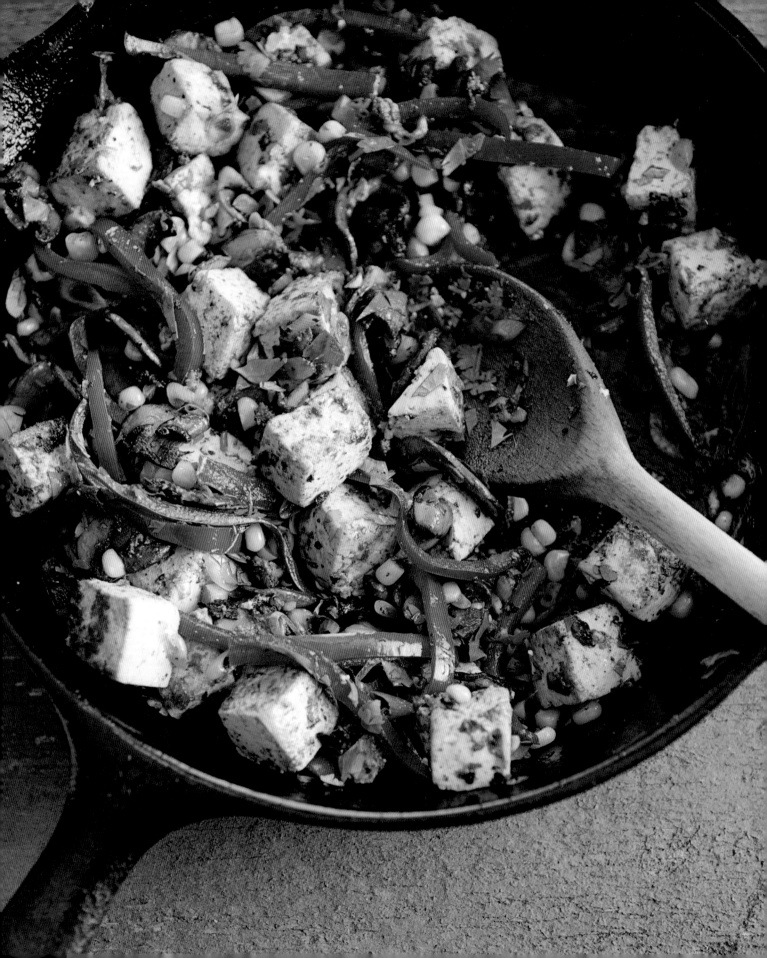

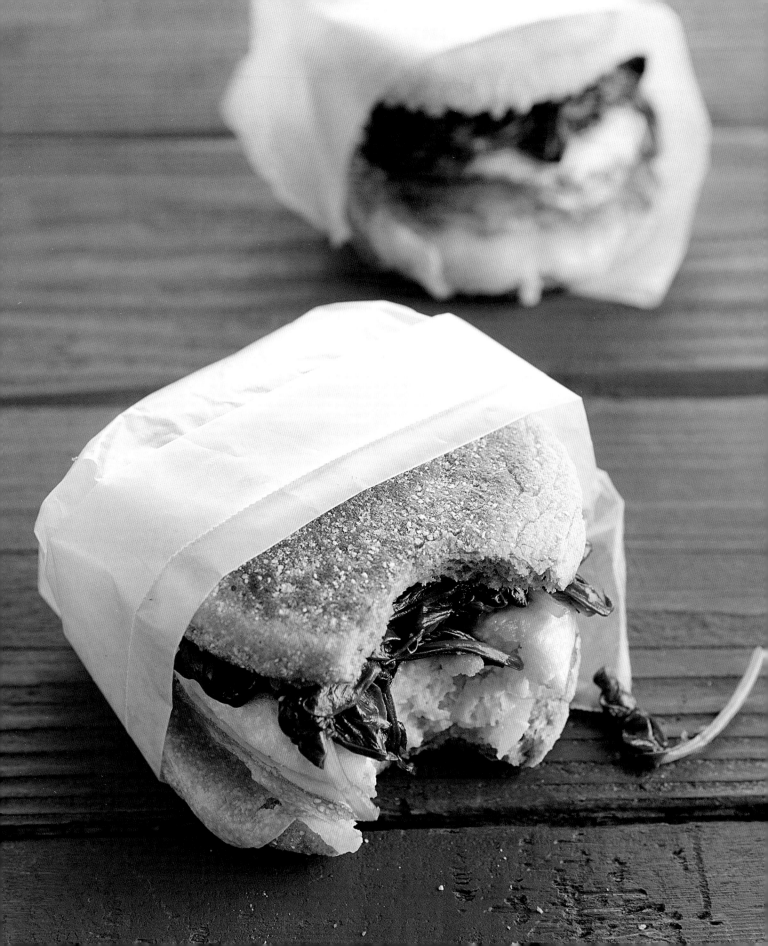

This egg sandwich is special enough for a weekend brunch, but quick enough to assemble for weekday mornings; baking the eggs instead of frying adds to the ease. If you don't have Manchego cheese, try using a sharp white Cheddar.

EGG SANDWICHES WITH WILTED SPINACH

olive oil, 1 tsp plus 1 Tbsp

large eggs, 2

low-fat (1%) milk or water, 2 Tbsp

Manchego cheese, 2 thin slices
(about 1½ oz/45 g total weight)

whole-wheat English muffins, 2, split
and toasted

garlic, 1 clove, smashed

baby spinach leaves, 2 generous
handfuls (about 3 oz/90 g)

MAKES 2 SANDWICHES

1 Preheat oven to 375°F (190°C). Lightly grease two 6-oz (185-g) ramekins with 1 teaspoon oil total.

2 In a bowl, scramble eggs lightly with milk. Divide mixture between ramekins. Bake just until eggs are puffy and set, 15–18 minutes.

3 Near end of baking time, place a cheese slice on bottom half of each toasted muffin. Place cheese-topped muffins on a rack in hot oven until cheese melts slightly, 2–3 minutes. Remove from oven and set aside.

4 Meanwhile, heat 1 tablespoon olive oil in a frying pan over medium heat and add garlic. Cook about a minute, just until garlic sizzles and is fragrant. Add spinach leaves and cook, stirring, just until wilted, 30 seconds–1 minute. Remove from heat and discard garlic clove.

5 Remove ramekins from oven and let cool slightly. Carefully run a paring knife around inside edges to release eggs. Turn out each egg portion onto a muffin, on top of melted cheese. Mound equal portions of spinach over eggs and then cover with muffin tops. Eat immediately, or wrap loosely in waxed paper and take to go.

This recipe is a lighter take on a fast-food favorite. To reduce the fat even more, omit the cheese and swap in 2 egg whites for 1 of the eggs.

eggs
- Source of high-quality protein
- Linked to weight loss when eaten for breakfast
- Source of choline, a nutrient needed for brain health

spinach
- Excellent source of folate, carotenoids, and vitamins A and K
- Helps protect against cancer
- Loaded with antioxidants

per sandwich 390 calories, 20 g protein, 31 g carbs, 21 g fat (7 g saturated fat), 205 mg cholesterol, 5 g fiber, 570 mg sodium

Tender, slightly bitter arugula gives a pleasant edge to the flavors of spicy–savory turkey sausage and nutty Parmesan cheese in this satisfying baked egg dish. Any leftovers make great sandwiches on whole–wheat bread with Dijon mustard.

FRITTATA WITH TURKEY SAUSAGE & ARUGULA

large eggs, 10

Parmesan cheese, ⅓ cup (1⅓ oz/40 g) freshly grated

low-fat (1%) milk, ¼ cup (2 fl oz/60 ml)

salt, ¼ tsp

freshly ground pepper, ¼ tsp

olive oil, 2 Tbsp

turkey sausages, 8 oz (250 g)

baby arugula, 4 cups packed (about 5 oz/155 g)

MAKES 8 SERVINGS

An easy way to reduce the cholesterol in this frittata is to substitute 4 egg whites for 2 of the eggs.

arugula
- From the cruciferous vegetable family, such as broccoli
- Good source of vitamin K
- Smaller leaves are milder in flavor than larger leaves

olive oil
- Rich in monounsaturated fats, which are linked to heart health
- Contains polyphenols that support healthy blood vessels and protect against cancer
- Linked to improved brain health

per serving
210 calories, 14 g protein, 2 g carbs, 16 g fat (4.5 g saturated fat), 280 mg cholesterol, 0 g fiber, 400 mg sodium

1 Preheat oven to 350°F (180°C).

2 In a large bowl, lightly whisk together eggs, cheese, milk, salt, and pepper. Set aside.

3 In a 10- or 12-inch (25- or 30-cm) ovenproof frying pan, heat 1 tablespoon of olive oil over medium-high heat. Turn sausages out of their casings into pan and cook, stirring constantly and breaking up meat into 1-inch (2.5-cm) pieces, until nicely browned on all sides, 3–4 minutes. Add arugula and stir just until evenly wilted, 1–2 minutes. Scrape sausage mixture into bowl with egg mixture.

4 Wipe pan clean and return to medium-high heat. Add remaining 1 tablespoon olive oil and spread to coat pan bottom. When oil is hot, pour egg mixture into pan and smooth top. Reduce heat to medium and cook, without stirring, for 1 minute.

5 Transfer pan to oven and bake until frittata is set in center and slightly puffed, 25–30 minutes. Let cool for 5 minutes in pan. Carefully run a paring knife or sharp-bladed spatula around inside edges to release frittata and slide onto a large plate. Cut frittata into wedges and serve warm or at room temperature.

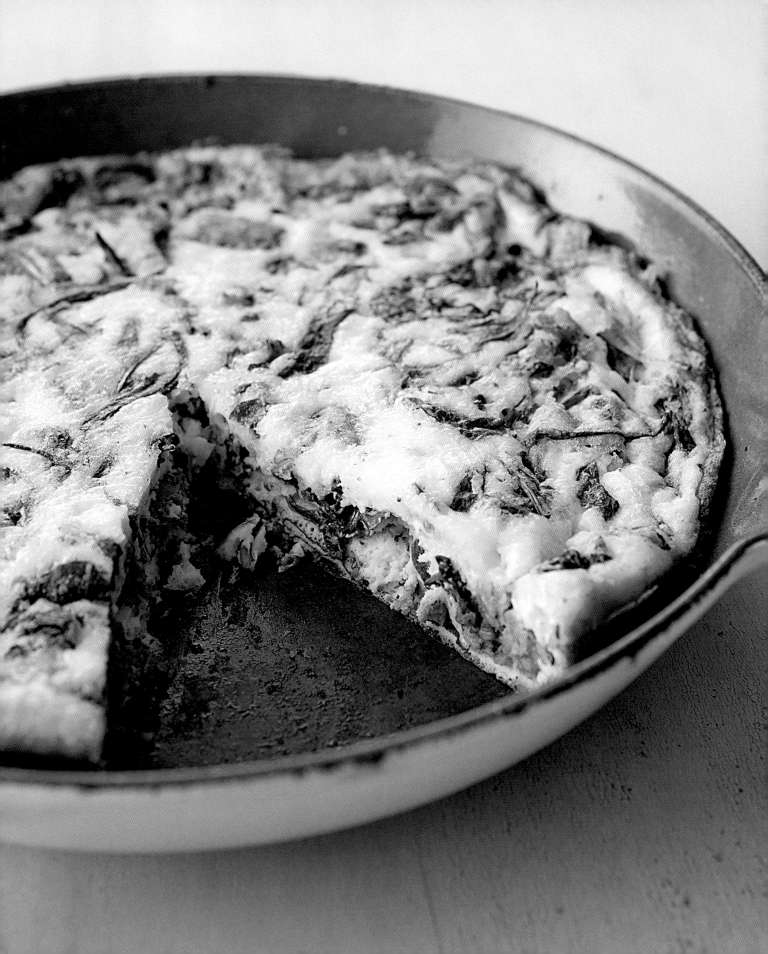

Toasted whole-wheat sourdough and a quick sauté of mushrooms and asparagus make a tasty bed for poached eggs. The key to poaching eggs is the timing, so watch carefully and remember that the egg will continue to cook a little after you remove it from the water.

POACHED EGGS WITH ASPARAGUS & MUSHROOMS

slender asparagus spears, 8

olive oil, 1 Tbsp

cremini mushrooms, 5 oz (155 g), sliced

garlic, 1 clove, pressed or minced

sea salt, ¼ tsp

freshly ground pepper, to taste

large eggs, 2

whole-wheat sourdough bread,
2 slices, toasted

MAKES 2 SERVINGS

Adding a good dose of vitamin-packed vegetables to your breakfast is a great way to start the day. Note that salting the poaching water will increase the recipe's sodium content.

asparagus

- Excellent source of vitamins A and K
- Contains fibers that improve digestive health
- Rich in anti-inflammatory compounds

mushrooms

- Believed to boost immunity
- Naturally low in calories
- Good source of potassium, selenium, and B vitamins

per serving 240 calories, 14 g protein, 19 g carbs, 13 g fat (3 g saturated fat), 185 mg cholesterol, 4 g fiber, 520 mg sodium

1 Break off and discard tough stem ends from asparagus. Cut spears on diagonal into 1¼-inch (3-cm) lengths. Set aside.

2 Heat olive oil in a nonstick frying pan over medium heat. Add mushrooms and asparagus and stir to coat with oil. Add garlic and cook, stirring, until garlic is fragrant but not browned, about 1 minute. Sprinkle with salt and pepper and cook, stirring often, until mushrooms are browned and asparagus is tender, 5–8 minutes. Remove from heat and set aside.

3 Bring a deep frying pan three-fourths full of lightly salted water to a boil over high heat. Adjust heat to maintain a simmer. Crack eggs, 1 at a time, into a measuring cup, and then gently slide into simmering water. Cook until eggs are softly set, about 3 minutes.

4 While eggs are cooking, arrange a slice of toast on each plate and make a bed of vegetable mixture on top of each toast, dividing it evenly. Using a slotted spoon, remove 1 egg at a time from pan, gently shaking off excess water and nestling atop each toast. Serve right away.

This fast Mexican scramble includes ripe tomatoes, mild green chiles, and corn tortilla strips that soften as they absorb the sauce, making it a hearty, flavorful breakfast. For extra color and an aromatic finish, top each serving with minced red onion and fresh cilantro leaves.

SCRAMBLED EGG CHILAQUILES

large eggs, 8

low-fat (1%) milk or water, 3 Tbsp

sea salt, a pinch

Cheddar cheese, ¼ cup
(1 oz/30 g) shredded

corn tortillas, 3

olive oil or vegetable oil, 2 Tbsp

large poblano chile, 1 (about 8 oz/250 g),
seeded and cut into thin strips

ripe tomatoes, 2, cored, seeded,
and chopped

MAKES 4 SERVINGS

1 In a bowl, beat eggs lightly with milk and salt until blended. Stir in shredded cheese. Set aside.

2 Stack tortillas and cut into quarters, then into thin strips. Set aside.

3 Heat olive oil in a large nonstick frying pan over medium heat. When oil is hot, add chile and cook, stirring often, until softened, 4–5 minutes. Add tortilla strips and cook, stirring constantly, until beginning to brown, about 2 minutes. Reduce heat to medium-low, add egg mixture, and cook, stirring often and scraping pan bottom to prevent sticking, until eggs are set but still soft and moist looking, 2–3 minutes longer. Gently stir in tomatoes and serve right away.

Here, corn tortillas are sautéed in heart-healthy olive oil for a lighter take on *chilaquiles*. For an egg scramble that's lower in cholesterol, swap in 8 egg whites for 4 of the eggs.

corn tortillas
- Rich in slowly digested complex carbs and fiber
- Can be compatible with a gluten-free diet

tomatoes
- Excellent source of vitamin C
- Contain the plant compound lycopene, which may protect against certain cancers
- Improve heart health by lowering cholesterol and preventing blood clots

per serving 290 calories,
16 g protein, 12 g carbs,
19 g fat (6 g saturated fat),
380 mg cholesterol, 2 g fiber,
230 mg sodium

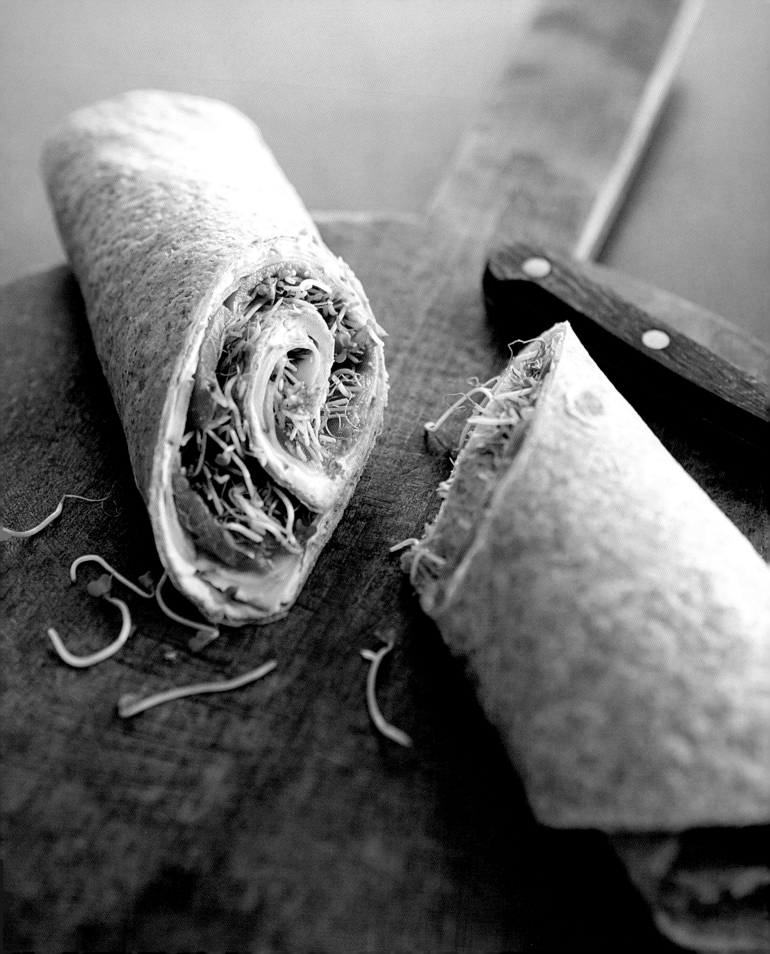

You can also serve this fast breakfast wrap as an eye-catching, light and healthy appetizer: double or triple the recipe and cut the wraps on the diagonal into 1½-inch (4-cm) slices. Look for sprouted-wheat tortillas at a natural-foods or well-stocked grocery store.

SMOKED SALMON & CUCUMBER WRAPS

sprouted-wheat or whole-wheat tortillas, 2 large

whipped light cream cheese, ¼ cup (2 oz/60 g)

English cucumber, ½ cup (2½ oz/75 g) very thinly sliced

smoked salmon, 2 oz (60 g), thinly sliced

broccoli sprouts or baby arugula leaves, 2 generous handfuls

MAKES 2 WRAPS

1 Spread each tortilla with half of cream cheese. Arrange half of cucumber slices on each in a single layer over cream cheese, overlapping them slightly if necessary and leaving a strip about 1 inch (2.5 cm) wide along one edge of tortilla uncovered. Arrange salmon over cucumbers, dividing it evenly. Scatter sprouts over cucumbers.

2 Roll up tortillas, beginning opposite the uncovered cream cheese and tucking tortilla snugly around ingredients. Press firmly on cream cheese end to seal. Turn seal side down and, using a serrated knife, cut each wrap in half on the diagonal. Serve right away or wrap tightly in waxed paper, plastic wrap, or aluminum foil and take to go.

Because smoked salmon is so flavorful, a little goes a long way. For a lower-sodium version, substitute poached or canned wild salmon.

salmon
- Excellent source of omega-3 fatty acids linked to brain and heart health
- Rich in vitamin D
- Promotes healthy eyes

broccoli sprouts
- Rich in powerful antioxidants
- Excellent source of vitamin K and selenium
- Good source of vitamin E

per wrap 210 calories, 11 g protein, 23 g carbs, 7 g fat (3.5 g saturated fat), 15 mg cholesterol, 3 g fiber, 950 mg sodium

These light bites don't just make your taste buds happy—they hold you over and keep your appetite in check, making it easier to eat moderately at the next mealtime.

SNACKS & STARTERS

QUICK-FIX IDEAS FOR SNACKS & STARTERS

PACK IT TO GO

EDAMAME Set a covered steamer over gently simmering water and add 1 cup (3 oz/90 g) fresh or frozen organic edamame (soybean) pods to the top part. Steam until the beans inside are tender, about 15 minutes. Drain the pods, then sprinkle with coarse sea salt. Let cool to room temperature and pack in a to-go container.

FRUITY SNACKS Cut up fresh fruit and add an unexpected ingredient for a new twist on a healthy snack. Try mango or watermelon chunks sprinkled with lime juice, chili powder, and sea salt; strawberries tossed with chopped fresh basil; or pineapple wedges with curry-spiked yogurt.

CUCUMBER-YOGURT DIP Stir together 1 container (7 oz/220 g) plain low-fat Greek yogurt, 1 cup (5 oz/155 g) grated or diced cucumber, a handful of chopped fresh mint or flat-leaf parsley, and a generous squeeze of fresh lemon juice in a to-go container. Season with salt and additional lemon juice, if needed. Pack with a bag of carrot sticks, bell pepper strips, or whole-wheat pita wedges.

MAKE IT AHEAD

SPICED NUTS Combine 2 parts each paprika and ground cumin with 1 part each brown sugar and coarse salt. Toss unsalted shelled almonds, cashews, pecans, or walnuts with a small amount of olive oil and the spice mixture to taste. Spread the nuts on a baking sheet and bake in a preheated 300°F (150°C) oven, shaking the sheet occasionally, until the nuts are fragrant, about 15 minutes. Let cool and store in an airtight container at room temperature for up to 1 week.

TRAIL MIX Visit the array of choices in the bulk-foods aisle to create a personalized trail mix. Mix together 4 or 5 different types of bite-sized superfoods (see pages 14–23) such as nuts like almonds, cashews, peanuts, or walnuts; dried fruit such as cherries, berries, apples, pineapple, and mango; and other nutritious ingredients like sunflower seeds, flaxseeds, pumpkin seeds, mini dark chocolate chips, and yogurt-covered raisins. Keep small containers of trail mix in your bag for a healthful snack anytime.

SERVE IT FOR COMPANY

GRILLED FRUIT Lightly grill sturdy fruits such as plum halves, mango slices, or pineapple wedges. Top with a small amount of strong-flavored cheese, such as crumbled Gorgonzola or feta.

WHITE BEAN CROSTINI Drain and rinse 1 can (15 oz/470 g) low-sodium cannellini or white kidney beans. Place the beans in a food processor along with 2 tablespoons olive oil, 2 teaspoons minced fresh sage, and 1 clove garlic, chopped. Purée until smooth, adding more olive oil if needed to achieve the desired consistency. Season to taste with salt and pepper and serve with toasted whole-grain baguette slices or whole-wheat crackers.

DRESSED-UP ASPARAGUS Bring a pot of salted water to a boil; meanwhile, trim a bunch of asparagus spears. Blanch the spears in the boiling water until bright green and crisp-tender, 2–4 minutes. Transfer to a bowl of ice water to stop the cooking. Drain and pat dry. Wrap thin strips of cured or smoked salmon around the spears and arrange on a platter. Sprinkle with finely grated lemon zest.

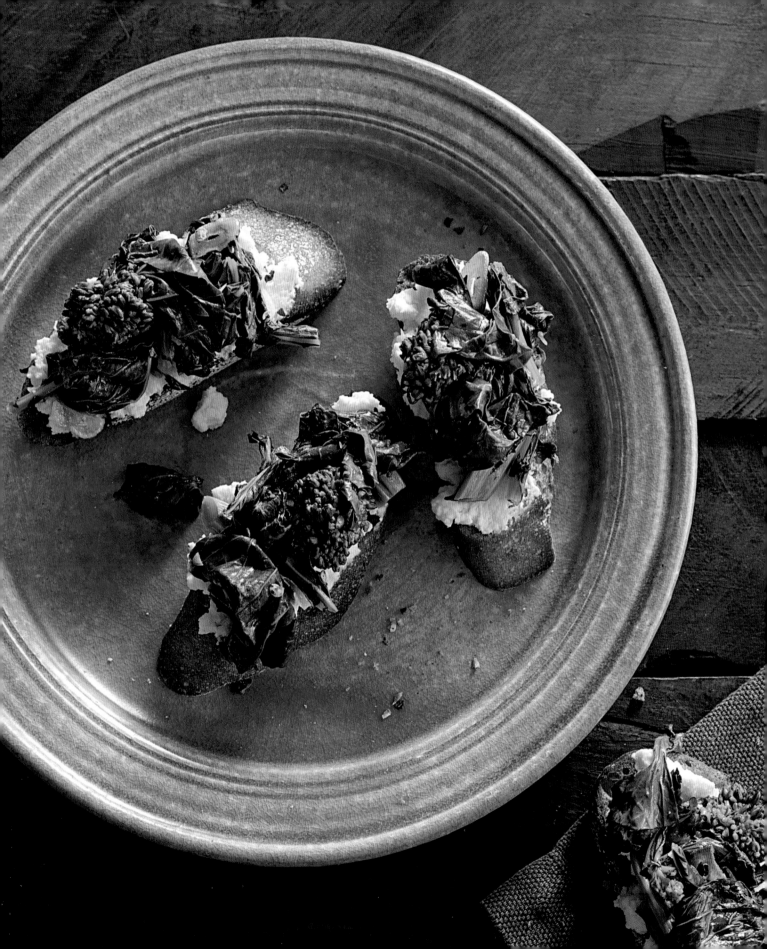

Broccoli rabe has a distinctively bitter flavor that goes well with the creamy cheese and pungent garlic. Substitute broccolini if you like a less bitter edge. You can make the topping a day ahead and refrigerate it; bring to room temperature before assembling the crostini.

BROCCOLI RABE & RICOTTA CROSTINI

whole-grain baguette, 1, cut on diagonal into 16 thin slices

extra-virgin olive oil, 3 Tbsp

garlic, 5 cloves, 2 left whole and 3 thinly sliced

part-skim ricotta cheese, 1 cup (8 oz/250 g)

broccoli rabe, 1 lb (500 g), ends trimmed

red pepper flakes, ¼ tsp

sea salt, ¼ tsp

MAKES 16 CROSTINI; 8 SERVINGS

1 Preheat oven to 375°F (190°C).

2 Arrange baguette slices on a baking sheet and toast in oven until crisp and lightly browned on edges, 10–12 minutes. Remove toasts from oven and let cool slightly.

3 Brush toasts lightly on one side with 1 tablespoon of olive oil total and scrape oiled sides using whole garlic cloves. Spread each slice with about 1 tablespoon of ricotta.

4 Coarsely chop broccoli rabe. Place in a colander and rinse well (do not dry). Heat remaining 2 tablespoons olive oil in a large frying pan over medium-high heat. Add sliced garlic and red pepper flakes and sauté until garlic is fragrant and just beginning to brown, about 30 seconds. Add broccoli rabe and salt and cook, stirring to coat broccoli rabe evenly with oil, until softened, about 2 minutes. Add 3 tablespoons water to pan, cover, and steam until liquid is evaporated and broccoli rabe is tender, 3–4 minutes. Remove from heat.

5 Spoon broccoli rabe mixture over ricotta on each crostini, dividing it evenly, and serve right away.

The combination of creamy ricotta, crunchy toasted bread, and garlicky, spicy greens gives these nutrient-rich snacks a decadent feel.

whole-grain bread
- Excellent source of energy-supplying complex carbs
- Whole grains are known to reduce the risk of stroke, heart disease, and type 2 diabetes

broccoli rabe
- High in vitamins A and K
- Good source of vitamin C and powerful antioxidants
- Contains compounds linked to cancer prevention

per serving 240 calories, 13 g protein, 27 g carbs, 10 g fat (2.5 g saturated fat), 10 mg cholesterol, 5 g fiber, 400 mg sodium

These refreshing rolls make perfect finger food for a spring or summer get-together; serve them with good-quality prepared chile and peanut dipping sauces (read the nutrition labels carefully before buying). Feel free to change up the filling ingredients as you please.

VEGETABLE SPRING ROLLS

You will swear off deep-fried egg rolls forever once you try these chewy, satisfying spring rolls, packed with fresh herbs and vegetables.

carrots

- Deep yellow-orange pigment is linked to reduced risk of cardiovascular disease
- May protect against colon cancer
- Excellent source of vitamin A

shiitake mushrooms

- Contain compounds that promote heart health
- Provide B vitamins, selenium, and potassium
- Believed to boost immunity

per roll 180 calories, 1 g protein, 32 g carbs, 5 g fat (.5 g saturated fat), 0 mg cholesterol, 3 g fiber, 25 mg sodium

shiitake mushrooms, ½ lb (250 g)
canola or peanut oil, 2 tsp
garlic, 1 clove, pressed or minced
low-sodium soy sauce, 1 tsp
thin dried rice noodles, 7 oz (220 g)
rice-paper wrappers, 12 (8½ inches/21.5 cm in diameter)
red bell pepper, 1, seeded and thinly sliced
ripe avocados, 2, pitted, peeled, and sliced
carrots, 2, peeled and cut into matchsticks
mixed fresh herb sprigs such as mint, cilantro, and basil, 1 cup packed (1 oz/30 g)

MAKES 12 ROLLS

1 Trim stems from shiitakes and discard (or save for soup or stock). Slice caps and set aside. In a large nonstick frying pan, heat 1½ teaspoons of oil over medium-high heat. Add garlic and cook, stirring, until fragrant but not browned, about 30 seconds. Add mushrooms and sauté until they have released their juices, 3–4 minutes. Add 1 teaspoon soy sauce and cook until pan is dry, about 1 minute. Transfer to a bowl and set aside.

2 Bring a pot of water to a boil over high heat. Add noodles, stir to separate, and cook until tender, 3–5 minutes or according to package directions. Drain in a colander and rinse under cold running water. Wipe pot dry, return noodles to pot, and toss with remaining ½ teaspoon oil.

3 Fill a large, shallow bowl with very hot tap water. Soak rice-paper wrappers, 1 or 2 at a time, until flexible, about 30 seconds. Shake off any excess water and stack on a plate. Place 1 wrapper flat on a work surface. Arrange a combination of noodles, bell pepper, avocado, mushrooms, carrots, and herbs across center of wrapper; fold ends in over filling, then roll up tightly from edge closest to you. Repeat to make more rolls.

4 Cut rolls in half on diagonal and serve right away.

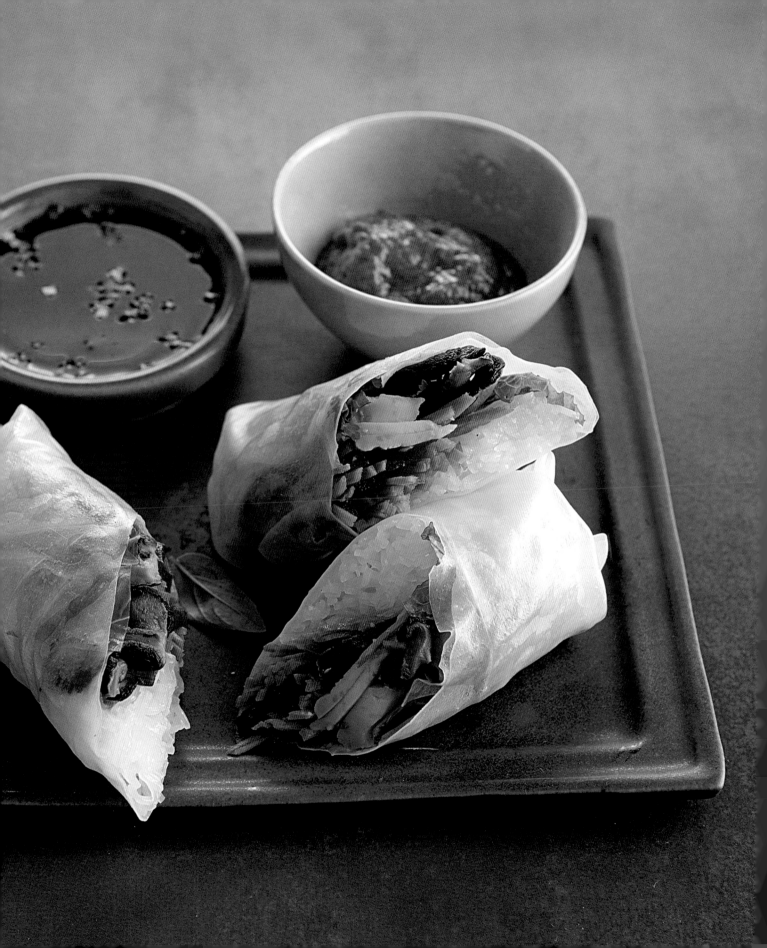

One of the easiest and most appealing of appetizers, tomato bruschetta comes together in minutes when you have ripe, juicy tomatoes on hand. Fresh mint adds an unexpected flash of flavor and fragrance, but you can substitute the classic fresh basil, if you like.

TOMATO & MINT BRUSCHETTA

Here, extra-virgin olive oil adds fruity flavor and helps your body absorb the fat-soluble lycopene found in tomatoes.

tomatoes
- High in lycopene, a plant compound believed to protect against heart disease and some types of cancer
- Good source of vitamins A and C and other antioxidants
- Rich in potassium

fresh mint
- Believed to aid digestion and stop the growth of certain harmful bacteria
- May help reduce inflammation associated with asthma

per serving 210 calories,
7 g protein, 34 g carbs,
4.5 g fat (1 g saturated fat),
0 mg cholesterol, 2 g fiber,
440 mg sodium

ripe tomatoes, preferably a combination of red and yellow, 1 lb (500 g)

extra-virgin olive oil, 2 Tbsp

sherry vinegar, 1 Tbsp

sea salt, ½ tsp

freshly ground pepper, to taste

baguette, 1, cut on diagonal into 16 thin slices

garlic, 1 clove, peeled but left whole

fresh mint, 2 Tbsp slivered

MAKES 16 TOASTS; 8 SERVINGS

1 Preheat oven to 350°F (180°C).

2 Core tomatoes and cut in half horizontally. Gently squeeze out seeds, using your fingertip to nudge them if necessary, and discard. Dice tomatoes and put in a bowl. Drizzle in 1 tablespoon of olive oil and vinegar and sprinkle with salt and pepper. Stir gently to mix. Set aside.

3 Arrange baguette slices on a baking sheet in a single layer and toast in oven until crisp and lightly browned on edges, about 15 minutes. Remove from oven and let cool slightly. Brush one side of each toast lightly with remaining 1 tablespoon olive oil and scrape oiled sides with garlic clove.

4 Mound tomato mixture on baguette slices, dividing evenly. Scatter a few slivers of mint on each. Arrange on a serving platter and serve right away.

Whole steamed artichokes make a simple, elegant appetizer or even side dish. If you whip up the dip and trim the artichokes while the water is coming to a boil, your work is done. Remember to set out an empty bowl for discarded leaves.

STEAMED ARTICHOKES WITH LEMONY YOGURT DIP

plain low-fat Greek yogurt, 1 cup (8 oz/250 g)

fresh lemon juice, 1 Tbsp plus ¼ cup (2 fl oz/60 ml)

paprika, ½ tsp

sea salt, ¼ tsp

freshly ground pepper, to taste

large globe artichokes, 4 (about 1 lb/500 g each)

MAKES 4 SERVINGS

1 In a bowl, stir together yogurt, 1 tablespoon lemon juice, paprika, salt, and pepper; set aside.

2 Bring a pot of water to a boil over high heat.

3 While water is heating, prepare artichokes: Trim stem ends and remove tough outer leaves around base. Using a sharp paring knife or vegetable peeler, remove fibrous peel from stems. Using a large, sharp knife, cut about 1 inch (2.5 cm) off tops of each artichoke.

4 Stir ¼ cup lemon juice into boiling water. Add artichokes and cook until base is tender when pierced with a knife, 20–25 minutes. Using tongs, remove from water and set aside until cool enough to handle. Carefully squeeze artichokes upside down to remove excess moisture.

5 Serve artichokes warm or at room temperature, with lemon-yogurt mixture on the side for dipping.

A dash of lemon juice and paprika turn rich Greek yogurt into a creamy dip for artichoke leaves, a healthy alternative to mayonnaise or melted butter.

artichokes
- Good source of fiber, folate, vitamin C, and magnesium
- Extremely rich in antioxidants
- Contain nutrients that promote liver health

greek-style yogurt
- Good source of calcium
- Contains beneficial bacteria that aid digestion
- Provides nearly three times the protein of traditional yogurt

per serving 120 calories, 9 g protein, 23 g carbs, 1.5 g fat (.5 g saturated fat), 0 mg cholesterol, 9 g fiber, 320 mg sodium

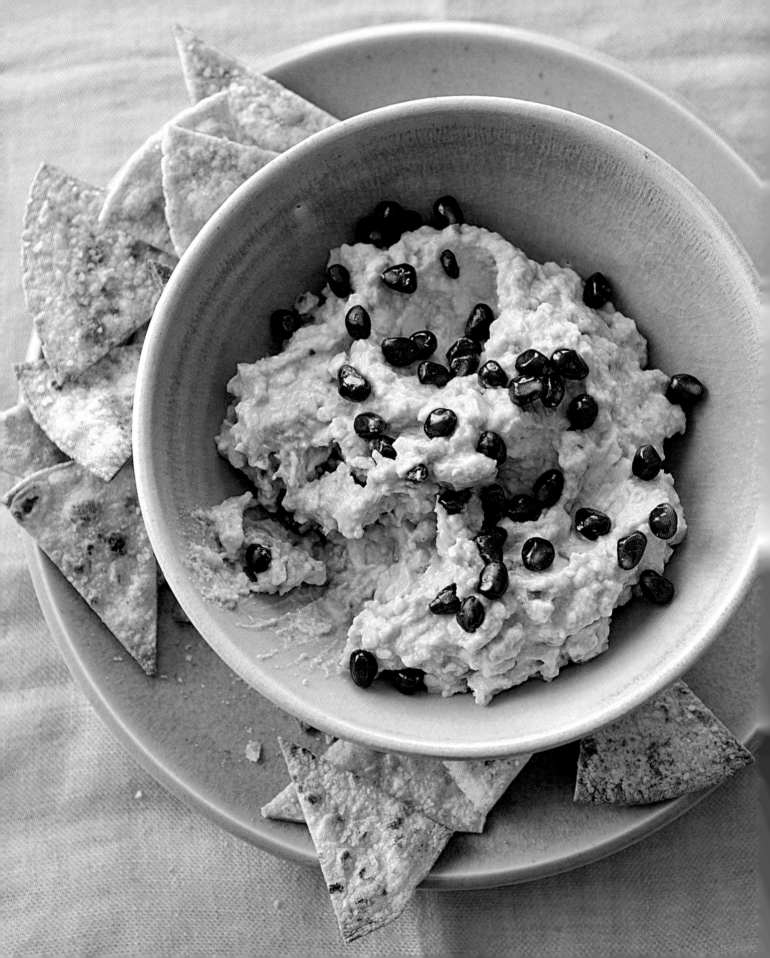

Fresh pomegranate seeds add a sweet, bright acidity and a splash of color to this classic guacamole. For the chips, seek out fresh, handmade corn tortillas, which are slightly thicker and more toothsome than the standard supermarket variety.

GUACAMOLE WITH BAKED CORN CHIPS

FOR CORN CHIPS
paprika, ¼ tsp
ground cumin, ¼ tsp
sea salt, ½ tsp
thick corn tortillas, 6
canola oil cooking spray

FOR GUACAMOLE
ripe avocados, 3
plain low-fat yogurt, ¼ cup (2 oz/60 g)

red onion, 3 Tbsp minced
fresh cilantro, 2 Tbsp chopped
fresh lime juice, 2 Tbsp
ground cumin, 1 Tbsp
garlic, 1 small clove, pressed or minced
jalapeño chile, 1–2 tsp seeded and minced
sea salt, ½ tsp
fresh pomegranate seeds, 3 Tbsp

MAKES 6 SERVINGS

1 Preheat oven to 375°F (190°C).

2 To make corn chips, in a small bowl, stir together paprika, cumin, and ½ teaspoon salt. Spray tortillas lightly on both sides with canola oil spray and sprinkle all sides with spice mixture. Stack tortillas and cut stack into 8 wedges. Arrange wedges in a single layer on a large baking sheet or sheets. Bake until chips are crisp and just starting to turn golden around edges, 10–15 minutes.

3 To make guacamole, cut avocados in half and remove pits. Scoop out flesh from peel and chop coarsely. Transfer to a bowl and mash with a fork to a chunky purée. Add yogurt, onion, cilantro, lime juice, cumin, garlic, jalapeño to taste, and ½ teaspoon salt and stir just until well combined. Taste and adjust seasonings.

4 Spoon guacamole into a serving bowl and top with pomegranate seeds. Serve right away with warm corn chips.

Packaged tortilla chips can be loaded with salt and fat; try baking your own chips instead, and whip up a batch of heart-healthy guacamole while they're in the oven.

avocados
- Excellent source of healthful monounsaturated fat
- Rich in cholesterol-lowering phytosterols
- Provide 20 essential nutrients

pomegranate seeds
- Rich in antioxidants linked to heart health and cancer prevention
- Good source of vitamin C and fiber

per serving 220 calories, 4 g protein, 23 g carbs, 14 g fat (2 g saturated fat), 0 mg cholesterol, 8 g fiber, 350 mg sodium

This is a great dip to make if you have a kitchen herb garden; swap in other fresh herbs such as thyme, tarragon, or basil. Serve it with a platter of raw vegetables for a tasty and beautiful appetizer. The dip can be prepared a day in advance and stored in the refrigerator.

CREAMY HERB DIP WITH CRUDITÉS

Low-fat yogurt enlivened with goat cheese and fresh herbs makes a rich-seeming, yet good-for-you dip for crunchy raw vegetables.

beets
- Rich in detoxifying compounds
- Excellent source of folate and manganese
- Contain antioxidants that protect against free radical damage

low-fat yogurt
- Rich in calcium and protein
- Contains nutrients that regulate blood pressure
- Look for "live active cultures" on the label

per serving 170 calories,
9 g protein, 21 g carbs,
6 g fat (3.5 g saturated fat),
10 mg cholesterol, 6 g fiber,
300 mg sodium

fresh goat cheese, 5 oz (155 g)
plain low-fat yogurt, ½ cup (4 oz/125 g)
fresh dill, 1 Tbsp chopped
fresh flat-leaf parsley, 1 Tbsp chopped
fresh lemon juice, 1 tsp
sea salt, ¼ tsp
freshly ground pepper, to taste

radishes, 3 large, thinly sliced
raw golden beets, 3 small, thinly sliced
sugar snap peas, ½ lb (250 g), trimmed
small carrots, 2 bunches, trimmed and peeled

MAKES ABOUT 1 CUP (8 OZ/250 G) DIP;
6 SERVINGS

1 In a blender or food processor, whirl goat cheese, yogurt, dill, parsley, and lemon juice until smooth. Season with salt and pepper. Transfer to a bowl.

2 Arrange radishes, beets, peas, and carrots on a platter. Place bowl of dip on platter and serve right away.

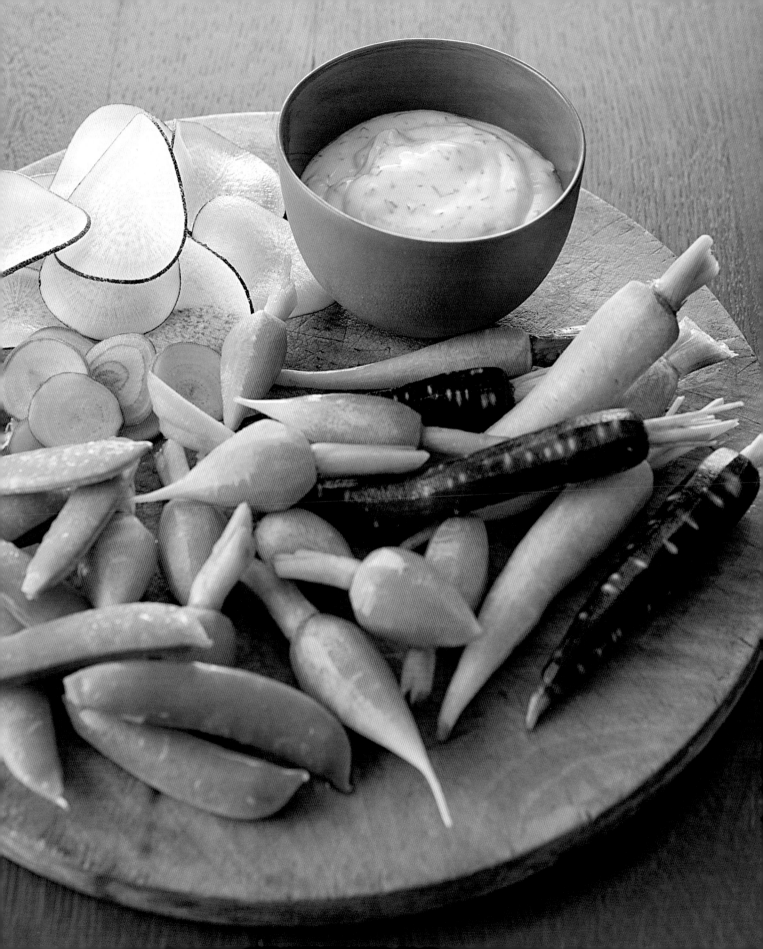

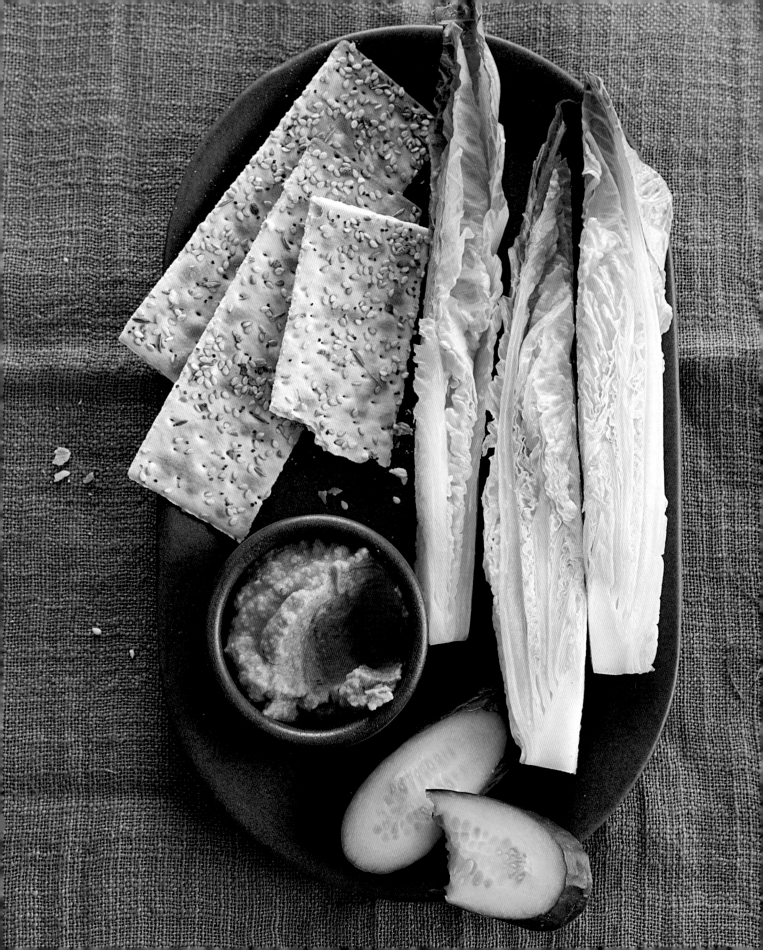

Roasted red pepper lends a sweet, smoky note and warm color to this classic chickpea dip, which is also delicious as a spread on sandwiches and wraps. Tahini, a purée of toasted sesame seeds, adds a subtle flavor, but if you don't have any around, feel free to leave it out.

ROASTED RED PEPPER HUMMUS

low-sodium chickpeas, 1 can (15 oz/470 g), drained and rinsed

roasted red bell pepper, 1, jarred or homemade (page 214), roughly chopped

olive oil, 2 Tbsp

tahini, 2 tsp

ground cumin, 1 tsp

smoked paprika, ½ tsp

sea salt, ½ tsp

fresh lemon juice, from 1 lemon

MAKES ABOUT 1 CUP (8 OZ/250 G); 6 SERVINGS

1 In a blender or food processor, whirl chickpeas, bell pepper, olive oil, tahini, cumin, paprika, salt, and lemon juice until smooth.

2 Serve right away, or transfer dip to an airtight container and refrigerate for up to 3 days.

This heart–healthy dip scores even more nutritional bonus points with the addition of puréed red bell pepper and ground sesame seeds.

chickpeas
- Protein and fiber help regulate blood sugar and control hunger
- Promote digestive health and help lower cholesterol
- Rich in heart-healthy nutrients

red bell peppers
- Excellent source of vitamins A and C
- Good source of folate, which supports heart health
- Contain cancer-fighting anti-inflammatory compounds

per serving 120 calories, 5 g protein, 15 g carbs, 9 g fat (1 g saturated fat), 0 mg cholesterol, 5 g fiber, 280 mg sodium

This summery salsa combines the sweet flavors of corn and edamame with tangy green tomatoes. Hulled tomatillos make a good substitute for the green tomatoes. Serve with Baked Corn Chips (page 65) or whole-grain crackers, or spoon over grilled fish or shrimp.

EDAMAME & GREEN TOMATO SALSA WITH CORN

Full of bright flavors, this out-of-the-ordinary salsa even packs some protein, thanks to the addition of edamame. Note that salting the cooking water will increase the sodium content of the dish.

edamame

- Rich in vegetable protein linked to heart health
- Contains the omega-3 fat alpha linolenic acid
- When possible, choose organic, non-genetically modified soybeans

per serving 60 calories, 3 g protein, 7 g carbs, 3 g fat (0 g saturated fat), 0 mg cholesterol, 2 g fiber, 80 mg sodium

shelled edamame (soybeans), 1 cup (5 oz/155 g)

sweet yellow corn kernels, from 1 large ear of corn (about ¾ cup/4 oz/125 g)

green tomatoes, ½ lb (250 g), cored

fresh lime juice, 2 Tbsp

olive oil, 1 Tbsp

red Fresno chile, 1, seeded and minced

red onion, ¼ cup (1½ oz/45 g) minced

fresh cilantro, 3 Tbsp chopped

salt, ¼ tsp

MAKES ABOUT 3 CUPS (18 OZ/560 G); 8 SERVINGS

1 Bring a saucepan of lightly salted water to a boil over high heat. Add edamame and corn and cook until just tender, 1–2 minutes. Drain in a colander and place under cold running water to cool. Drain again and set aside until needed.

2 Put tomatoes in a food processor and pulse just until coarsely chopped. Transfer to a large bowl and stir in edamame, corn, lime juice, olive oil, chile, onion, cilantro, and salt. Serve right away, or cover and refrigerate for up to 4 hours. Bring to room temperature before serving.

Toasted and spiced nuts make a perfect party nibble or super-portable snack. This rendition yields nuts that are both spicy and tangy, thanks to the lime juice. You can also experiment with other flavor combinations, such as sesame oil and honey or soy sauce and wasabi.

CHILI-LIME ALMONDS

whole raw almonds, 1½ cups
(6 oz/185 g)

fresh lime juice, 3 Tbsp

olive oil or canola oil, 1 tsp

chili powder, 1 tsp

sea salt, ½ tsp

light brown sugar, ½ tsp firmly packed

cayenne pepper, ¼ tsp

MAKES 1½ CUPS (6 OZ/185 G);
6 SERVINGS

1 Preheat oven to 300°F (150°C).

2 Spread almonds in a single layer on a baking sheet and toast in oven until lightly browned and fragrant, about 15 minutes.

3 Meanwhile, in a bowl, stir together lime juice, oil, chili powder, salt, brown sugar, and cayenne. Add hot almonds to bowl straight from oven and stir to coat thoroughly. Leave oven on and reserve pan.

4 Let nuts stand for about 5 minutes, stirring again every minute or so. Drain any remaining liquid and return almonds to baking sheet. Bake until golden brown and dry, 8–10 minutes longer. Let cool completely on pan. Store in an airtight container at room temperature for up to 1 week.

Loaded with fiber and protein, these flavorful nuts will give you a welcome boost of energy.

almonds
- Rich in heart-smart nutrients like mono- and polyunsaturated fats, potassium, and vitamin E
- Nuts are a good source of vegetarian protein
- Almonds with skins on have the most nutritional value

cayenne pepper
- Known to have anti-inflammatory and pain-relief properties
- Enhances immunity, metabolism, and heart health

per serving 220 calories, 8 g protein, 9 g carbs, 18 g fat (1.5 g saturated fat), 0 mg cholesterol, 5 g fiber, 200 mg sodium

These crispy baked chips made from sturdy fresh greens are every bit as addictive as other chips, but guilt-free. The secret to turning out perfect kale chips is to distribute the oil and spices evenly on the leaves, and to avoid overcrowding them on the baking sheet.

KALE CHIPS WITH SEA SALT & SMOKED PAPRIKA

curly or dinosaur kale, 1 bunch (½ lb/250 g)

olive oil, 2 Tbsp

smoked paprika, ¼ tsp

coarse sea salt, ½ tsp

MAKES 4 SERVINGS

Rather than heading for the chip aisle in search of a crunchy snack, veer toward the produce section—these baked vegetable chips will satisfy your craving.

kale

- Source of antioxidants known to prevent cancer and promote eye health and detoxification
- Excellent source of vitamins A, C, and K
- Provides an easily absorbed form of calcium

per serving 90 calories, 2 g protein, 6 g carbs, 7 g fat (1 g saturated fat), 0 mg cholesterol, 1 g fiber, 270 mg sodium

1 Preheat oven to 300°F (150°C).

2 Rinse kale well and blot dry thoroughly with a clean kitchen towel. Tear leaves from ribs; discard ribs. Using your hands, tear leaves into fairly large, appealing chip-size pieces.

3 Place kale in a bowl and sprinkle with olive oil, paprika, and salt. Using your hands, toss to coat evenly with oil and seasoning.

4 Arrange leaves in a single layer on 2 baking sheets. Bake, rotating pans top to bottom and back to front midway through baking time, until leaves are dry and crispy, about 25 minutes. Serve right away; kale chips are best eaten within a few hours.

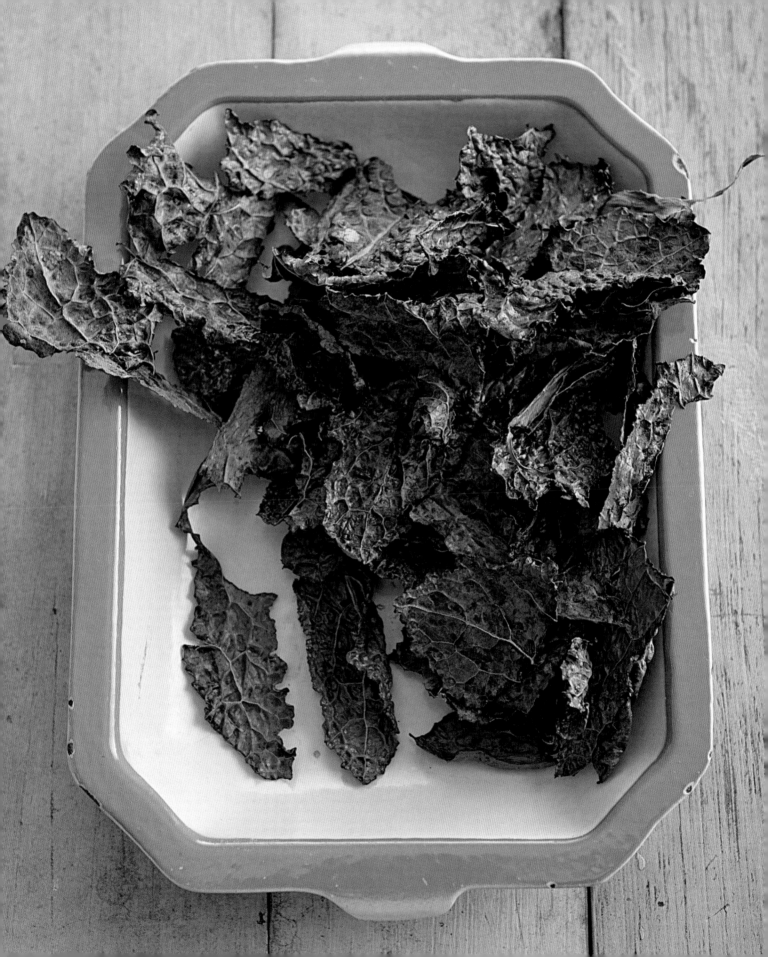

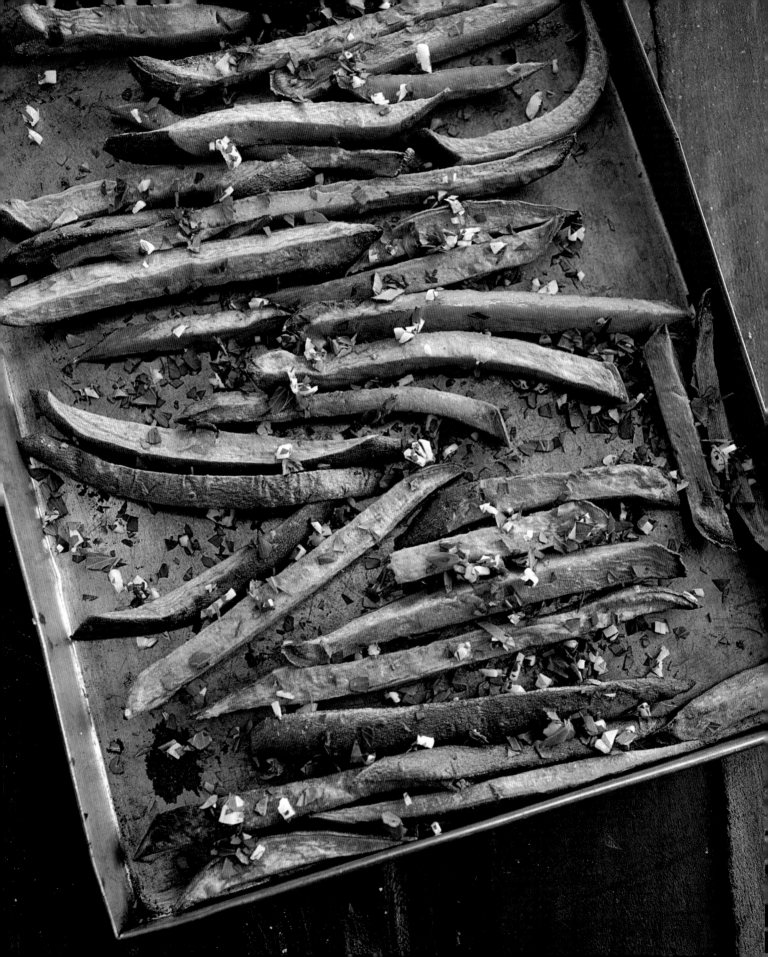

Serve these enticing oven fries as an after-school snack or a side dish—they go equally well with sandwiches and turkey burgers or roast chicken and fish. Use organic sweet potatoes, if possible, since they are not peeled. If you're not a fan of raw garlic, feel free to omit it.

SWEET POTATO OVEN FRIES

orange-fleshed sweet potatoes,
2 lb (1 kg)
olive oil, 2 Tbsp
coarse sea salt, ¼ tsp
Parmesan cheese, 3 Tbsp freshly grated
fresh flat-leaf parsley, 2 Tbsp chopped
garlic, 1 clove, minced
MAKES 6 SERVINGS

1 Preheat oven to 450°F (230°C).

2 Scrub, rinse, and dry sweet potatoes; do not peel. Cut lengthwise into slices ½ inch (12 mm) thick, then cut each slice into batons about ¼ inch (6 mm) wide and 3 inches (7.5 cm) long.

3 Pile potatoes on a large rimmed baking sheet and toss with olive oil and salt. Spread in pan in a single layer. Roast, stirring with a heatproof spatula midway through baking time, until tender and edges are nicely browned, 20–25 minutes.

4 In a large bowl, stir together Parmesan, parsley, and garlic until well mixed. Add fries and toss gently to coat. Serve right away.

Nutrient-dense sweet potato fries are a healthy alternative to standard French fries, and chances are they will get devoured just as quickly.

sweet potatoes
- Packed with beta-carotene and vitamin A
- Rich in fiber and potassium linked to heart health
- Pair with healthy fats such as olive oil to enhance absorption of many of their nutrients

parmesan cheese
- Excellent source of calcium
- Strongly flavored, so you need less than other cheeses, reducing overall fat and sodium

per serving 180 calories,
4 g protein, 31 g carbs,
5 g fat (1 g saturated fat),
0 mg cholesterol, 5 g fiber,
210 mg sodium

These homemade bars make great snacks or lunch-box treats. You can assemble them in minutes and walk away while they set in the refrigerator; no baking required! Use this recipe as a template for variations using any of your favorite dried fruits and nuts.

CHEWY FRUIT & NUT BARS

A host of healthy ingredients make up these bars, which are infinitely better than packaged granola bars because you know exactly what's in them.

cashews
- Lower fat content than most other nuts
- High percentage of heart-healthy monounsaturated fat
- Excellent source of magnesium

dried apricots
- Excellent source of potassium
- High in beta-carotene and vitamin A
- Choose unsulfured if available

per bar 170 calories,
3 g protein, 20 g carbs,
9 g fat (1.5 g saturated fat),
0 mg cholesterol, 2 g fiber,
40 mg sodium

unsalted butter, 1 tsp plus 2 Tbsp

puffed brown rice cereal, 1½ cups (6 oz/185 g)

whole almonds, 1 cup (4 oz/125 g)

whole cashews, ½ cup (3 oz/90 g)

dried cranberries, 1 cup (4 oz/125 g)

dried apricots, ½ cup (3 oz/90 g) chopped

brown rice syrup, ½ cup (5 oz/155 g)

unsalted creamy almond butter, ¼ cup (2½ oz/75 g)

light brown sugar, 2 Tbsp firmly packed

salt, ¼ tsp

MAKES 20 BARS

1 Line an 8-inch (20-cm) square baking pan with aluminum foil, leaving an inch or so of overhang on 2 opposite edges to use later as a handle. Grease foil with 1 teaspoon butter.

2 In a large bowl, stir together brown rice cereal, almonds, cashews, cranberries, and apricots. Set aside.

3 In a saucepan over medium heat, stir or whisk together brown rice syrup, almond butter, brown sugar, 2 tablespoons butter, and salt until mixture is smooth. Bring to a simmer and cook for 1 minute, stirring constantly to prevent scorching.

4 Immediately pour hot almond-butter mixture over cereal mixture in bowl. Using a wooden spoon, mix until cereal, fruit, and nuts are evenly coated and distributed.

5 With lightly buttered hands, press mixture firmly and evenly into prepared pan. Refrigerate until set, about 1 hour. Lift out of pan and transfer to a cutting board. Use a sharp buttered knife to cut into 20 small bars; remove from foil. Store in refrigerator in an airtight container, with sheets of waxed paper between layers, for up to 1 week.

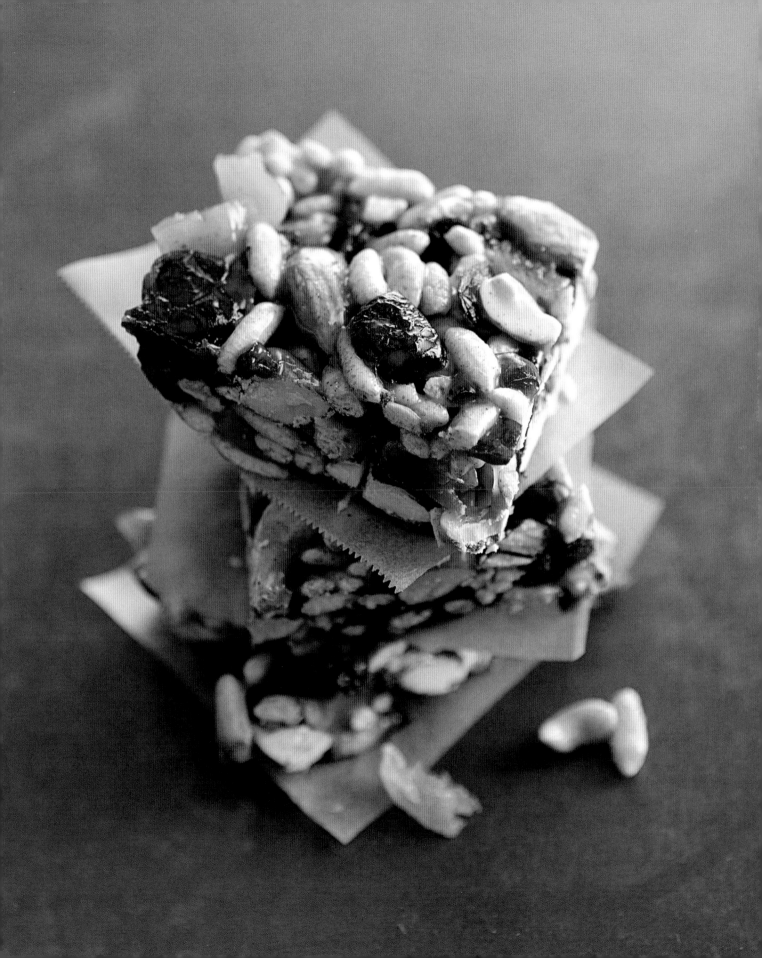

Taking a break for a midday meal gives you the chance to relax and refuel. Choosing foods like whole grains and lean protein can provide nutrients to help you focus and think clearly all afternoon long.

LUNCH

QUICK-FIX IDEAS FOR LUNCH

EAT IT ON THE RUN

PROTEIN WRAP Spread Roasted Red Pepper Hummus (page 69) on a whole-wheat tortilla. Top with shredded carrots or beets, shredded hard-boiled egg, and a dash or two of hot sauce, and season lightly with salt and pepper. Fold in two sides of the tortilla and then roll it up like a burrito; wrap in foil or plastic wrap and eat out of hand.

FARMER'S SANDWICH Spread the cut side of a whole-wheat roll with grainy mustard. Spread the other half with prepared onion jam or tomato chutney. Top with low-fat sharp Cheddar cheese slices, thin apple slices, and a few baby spinach leaves. Place in a sandwich bag, or wrap in foil or plastic wrap, and eat out of hand.

TOMATO-BASIL PITAS Stuff a whole-wheat pita pocket with fresh mozzarella slices, tomato slices, chopped roasted red peppers, baby arugula leaves, and basil leaves. Drizzle with a little balsamic vinegar and sprinkle with salt. Wrap in foil or plastic wrap and eat out of hand (don't let the pita sit for too long or it will get soggy).

PACK IT TO GO

BEAN & TUNA SALAD Combine 2 parts cooked low-sodium white beans or chickpeas and 1 part canned, flaked water-packed tuna in a to-go container. Add halved cherry tomatoes, minced red onion, and chopped fresh parsley. Drizzle with olive oil and fresh lemon juice, add a small spoonful of grainy mustard, and season lightly with salt and pepper. Cover and shake the ingredients well to combine.

GRAPEFRUIT & AVOCADO SALAD Combine shaved green cabbage or napa cabbage, grapefruit sections, avocado slices, and fresh cilantro leaves in a to-go container. Drizzle with olive oil and fresh lime juice, season with salt and pepper, and garnish with toasted pumpkin seeds. Cover and shake gently to combine.

JAPANESE-STYLE RICE BOWL Fill a to-go container about halfway with cooked brown rice. Add a splash of rice vinegar and a generous sprinkle of toasted sesame seeds and stir to combine. Top the rice with ingredients of your choice, such as thin strips of nori (dried seaweed), chopped green onion, cooked spinach or broccoli, snow peas, shelled edamame (soybeans), or cooked tofu. Pack with a packet of low-sodium soy sauce. Eat at room temperature or slightly warmed in a microwave.

MAKE IT AHEAD

ROASTED RED PEPPERS Broil a couple of red bell peppers, turning as needed, until the skins are blistered and the peppers are soft, 10–15 minutes (see page 214). Let cool, then peel, remove the seeds, and slice into strips. Transfer the strips and any juices to a jar and add 2 tablespoons olive oil and 1 clove garlic, minced. Stir to combine. Cover and store in the refrigerator for up to 1 week. Add roasted pepper strips to sandwiches, wraps, or grain salads.

COOKED QUINOA Bring 2 parts water or low-sodium broth to a boil, add 1 part rinsed quinoa, and reduce the heat to low. Cover and simmer until the grains are tender, about 15 minutes. Let cool, then transfer to an airtight container and store in the refrigerator for up to 4 days. Use quinoa to bulk up your favorite lunch salad, or combine it with olive oil, vinegar, and chopped vegetables and fresh herbs for a hearty grain salad.

POACHED CHICKEN Bring a large saucepan of water to a boil over high heat. Add ½ teaspoon salt and 2 or 3 boneless, skinless chicken breast halves. Reduce the heat until the water is barely simmering and cook until the chicken is just opaque in the center, 8–10 minutes. Transfer to a plate or cutting board to cool. Store in an airtight container in the refrigerator for up to 4 days. Shred or chop as needed for salads, wraps, or sandwiches.

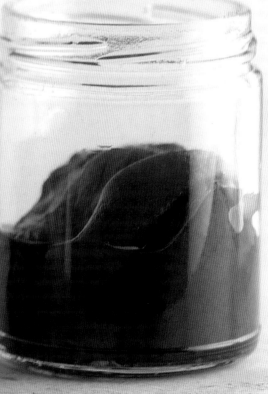

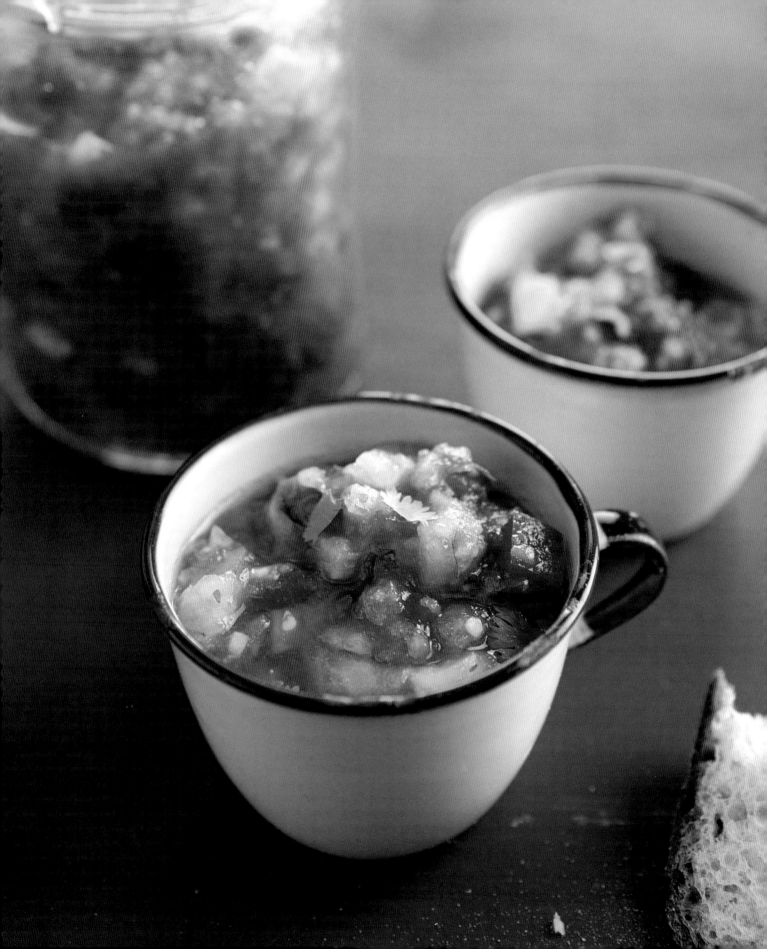

This recipe calls for heirloom tomatoes, which come in a wide range of colors and have a much-deserved reputation for knockout flavor. For a heartier meal, garnish each serving with a couple of grilled shrimp (page 131) and serve with crusty bread.

HEIRLOOM TOMATO GAZPACHO

ripe heirloom tomatoes, 2½ lb (1.25 kg), cored and cut into chunks

low-sodium tomato juice, ¾ cup (6 fl oz/180 ml), plus more if needed

fresh lime juice, 3 Tbsp

red wine vinegar, 1 Tbsp

red bell pepper, 1, seeded and diced

English cucumber, ⅓ cup (2 oz/60 g) diced

garlic, 1 clove, minced

jalapeño chile, 1 small, seeded and minced

fresh cilantro, 2 Tbsp chopped

sea salt, ⅛ tsp

MAKES 4 SERVINGS

1 In a blender or food processor, coarsely purée tomatoes, a portion at a time. Pour into a large bowl.

2 Stir in ¾ cup (6 fl oz/180 ml) tomato juice, lime juice, and vinegar until well blended. Add bell pepper, cucumber, garlic, jalapeño, cilantro, and salt and stir gently until evenly distributed. Add up to ½ cup (4 fl oz/125 ml) more tomato juice to thin soup to desired consistency, if necessary.

3 Serve soup at room temperature or chill until cold, about 1 hour. Ladle into bowls and serve right away.

Taste the soup before adding salt—you might find that you don't need it. Better yet, pump up the flavor by adding more lime juice, vinegar, or cilantro.

tomatoes
- High in lycopene, which is thought to protect against cancer and heart disease
- Good source of vitamins A and C, as well as other antioxidants
- Source of fiber and potassium

vinegar
- Adds flavor without adding extra calories
- Shown to help decrease calorie intake by helping to regulate blood sugar

per serving 80 calories, 3 g protein, 17 g carbs, .5 g fat (0 g saturated fat), 0 mg cholesterol, 5 g fiber, 115 mg sodium

This fall-inspired soup comes together quickly when you use precut squash, available fresh in many supermarkets, and an immersion blender to blend the soup in the pot. If you have a lot of squash, make a double batch of the soup and freeze for up to 3 months.

BUTTERNUT SQUASH & APPLE SOUP WITH PUMPKIN SEEDS

Loaded with vitamins and minerals, this wholesome soup gets a topping of low-fat yogurt and energy-boosting seeds.

butternut squash
- Excellent source of vitamin A and beta-carotene, powerful antioxidants
- Provides vitamin C and fiber
- Ample amount of potassium helps regulate blood pressure

pumpkin seeds
- Rich source of minerals such as iron and zinc
- Excellent source of magnesium, shown to regulate blood sugar
- Linked to men's prostate and bone health

per serving 210 calories, 5 g protein, 36 g carbs, 7 g fat (1.5 g saturated fat), 0 mg cholesterol, 6 g fiber, 190 mg sodium

olive oil, 2 Tbsp

yellow onion, 1, thinly sliced

sea salt, ½ tsp

garlic, 1 clove, pressed or minced

water or low-sodium chicken or vegetable broth or stock, 4 cups (32 fl oz/1 l)

butternut squash, about 3 lb (1.5 kg), peeled, seeded, and cut into cubes (about 9 cups)

tart apples such as Granny Smith, 2, peeled, cored, and chopped

freshly grated nutmeg, ¼ tsp

plain low-fat yogurt, 6 Tbsp (3 oz/90 g)

toasted pumpkin seeds, 2 Tbsp

MAKES 6 SERVINGS

1 Heat olive oil in a large pot over medium heat. Add onion and salt and sauté until onion is softened and beginning to brown, 4–6 minutes. Add garlic and cook, stirring constantly, until softened and fragrant but not browned, about 1 minute longer.

2 Add water, squash, apples, and nutmeg. Raise heat to high and bring to a boil. Reduce heat to maintain a simmer, cover, and cook, stirring occasionally, until squash is tender when pierced with a fork, about 20 minutes. Remove from heat and let cool slightly.

3 Using an immersion blender in the pot, purée soup until smooth. Or, transfer soup, in batches if necessary, to a blender or food processor and purée until smooth; return to pot and reheat if necessary. Ladle soup into bowls and top each serving with about 1 tablespoon yogurt and 1 teaspoon pumpkin seeds. Serve hot.

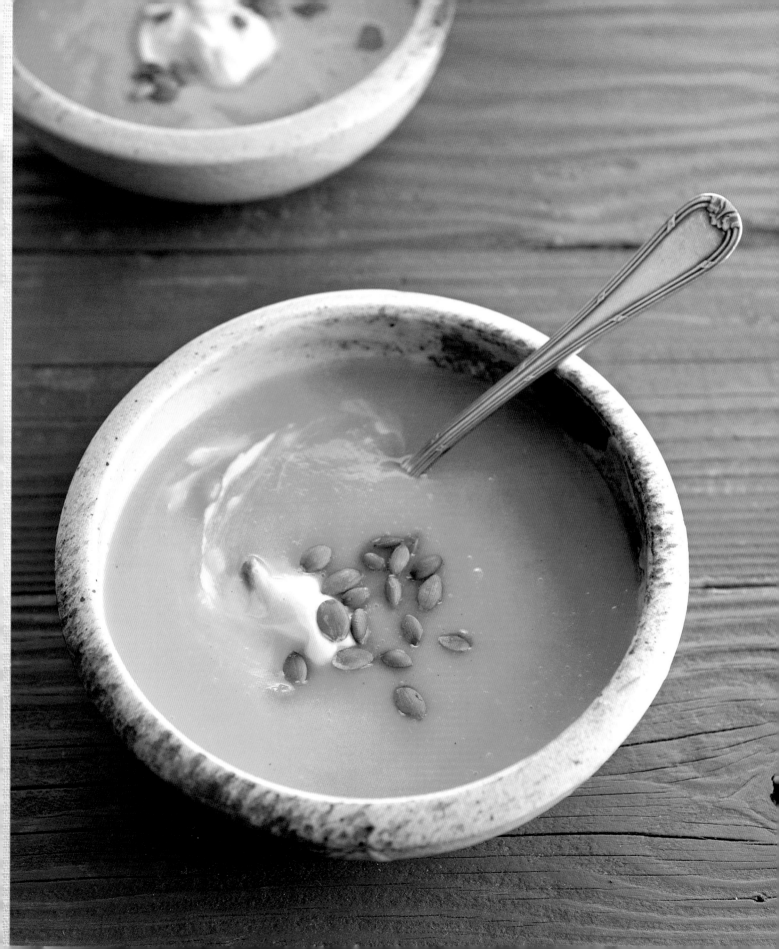

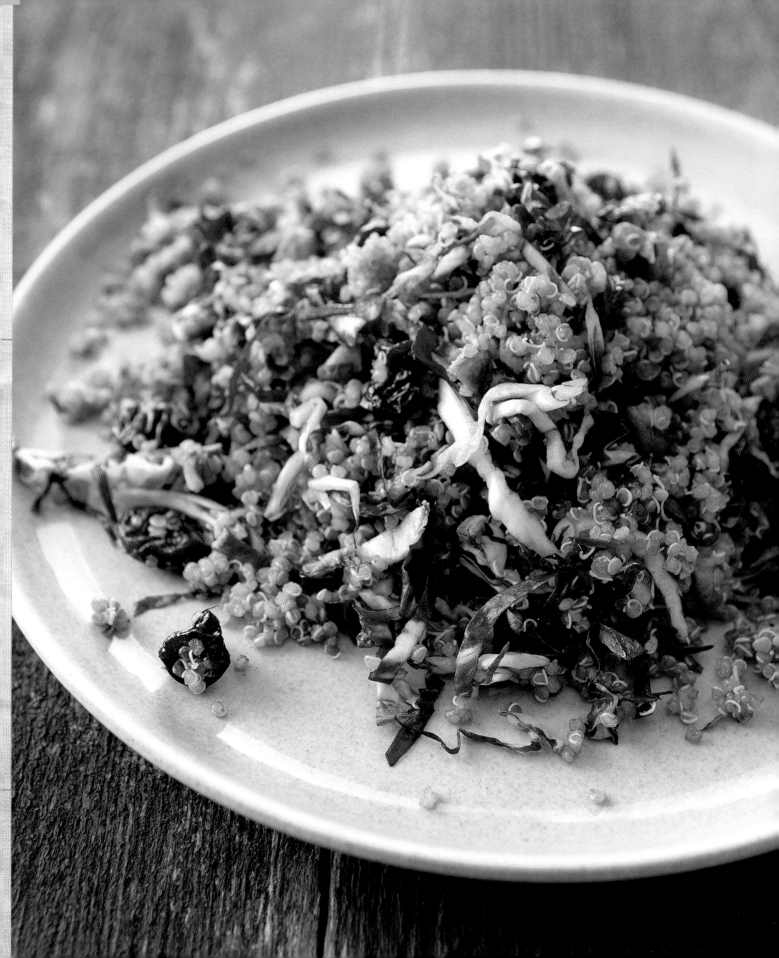

Once you start using quinoa in salads, chances are you'll get hooked; it is a no-fuss grain that is extremely forgiving to cook, yielding tender pearls full of nutty flavor. Use this recipe as a starting point, swapping in other fresh ingredients such as kale, corn, and cilantro.

QUINOA SALAD WITH DRIED CHERRIES & PISTACHIOS

quinoa, 1 cup (8 oz/250 g)
radicchio, ½ head (about 4 oz/125 g), cored and thinly sliced
balsamic vinegar, ¼ cup (2 fl oz/60 ml)
extra-virgin olive oil, 2 Tbsp
dried tart cherries, ¼ cup (1 oz/30 g)

pistachios, ¼ cup (1 oz/30 g), chopped
fresh flat-leaf parsley, 3 Tbsp chopped
sea salt, ¼ tsp
freshly ground pepper, to taste

MAKES 4 SERVINGS

1 Put quinoa in a fine-mesh strainer and rinse well under cold water. In a saucepan, bring 2 cups (16 fl oz/500 ml) water to a boil over high heat. Add quinoa and reduce heat to low. Cover and simmer until grains are tender and water is absorbed, about 15 minutes. Remove quinoa from heat and let cool slightly. Transfer to a large bowl and fluff with a fork to separate grains.

2 Add radicchio, vinegar, olive oil, cherries, pistachios, and parsley to bowl with warm quinoa and stir to mix well. Season with salt and pepper. Serve warm or at room temperature.

This flavorful, protein-rich salad will provide a welcome energy boost to get you through a late-afternoon slump.

dried tart cherries
- Loaded with antioxidants
- Reduce inflammation associated with heart disease and arthritis
- Choose unsulfured if available

pistachios
- One of the lowest calorie, highest protein nuts
- Promotes satiety, helping you eat less overall
- Rich source of vitamin B6 to help regulate mood and promote brain health

per serving 310 calories, 8 g protein, 41 g carbs, 13 g fat (1.5 g saturated fat), 0 mg cholesterol, 4 g fiber, 160 mg sodium

For an elegant fall lunch, serve this colorful salad with butternut squash soup (page 84). Slice and add the pears just before serving, as the flesh will brown very quickly. Avoid painstaking prep by purchasing fresh pomegranate seeds at the market.

SPINACH, PEAR & POMEGRANATE SALAD

Pomegranate seeds and walnuts add extra antioxidant power to this seriously nutritious—and delicious—salad.

spinach
- Good source of folate and carotenoids
- Rich in vitamins and minerals
- Linked to blood clotting and bone and eye health

pears
- The fruit's high water content promotes fullness
- High in fiber
- Promote heart health and digestive function

per serving 260 calories, 6 g protein, 26 g carbs, 16 g fat (3 g saturated fat), 5 mg cholesterol, 5 g fiber, 350 mg sodium

walnut pieces, ⅓ cup (1½ oz/45 g)

cider vinegar, 3 Tbsp

extra-virgin olive oil, 2 Tbsp

honey, 1 Tbsp

Dijon mustard, 1 tsp

salt, ¼ tsp

freshly ground pepper, ⅛ tsp

baby spinach, 8 oz (250 g)

ripe pears such as Bartlett, 2, cored and sliced

pomegranate seeds, ½ cup (2½ oz/75 g)

blue cheese, ¼ cup (1¼ oz/37 g) crumbled

MAKES 4 SERVINGS

1 Preheat oven to 350°F (180°C). Spread walnuts on a baking sheet and toast in oven until lightly browned and fragrant, about 10 minutes. Immediately pour onto a plate to cool. Set aside.

2 In a large bowl, whisk together vinegar, olive oil, honey, mustard, salt, and pepper to make a dressing.

3 Add spinach, pears, pomegranate seeds, and walnuts to bowl and toss gently to mix and coat well. Divide salad among 4 plates or bowls and top each with about 1 tablespoon blue cheese. Serve right away.

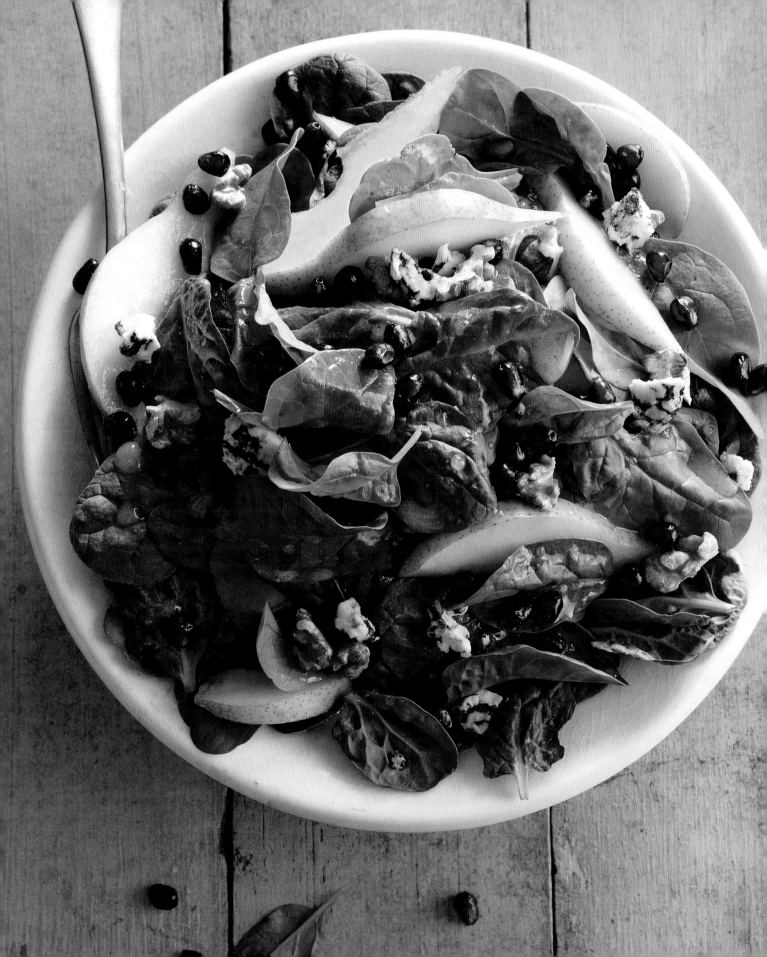

Letting the salad sit for a few minutes will allow the flavors to meld and the croutons to soften a bit, but don't let it sit for too long or the ingredients will grow soggy. As a shortcut to making the croutons, you can simply spoon the salad into warmed pita pockets.

GREEK CHICKEN SALAD WITH PITA CROUTONS

The Mediterranean diet is one of the healthiest in the world, and this salad draws on many typical ingredients from that region, including cucumbers, tomatoes, and olive oil.

cucumbers
- Have been linked to a clear complexion
- A natural diuretic

chicken breast
- Quick-cooking lean protein
- Excellent source of B vitamins
- Removing skin can substantially reduce fat

per serving 380 calories, 37 g protein, 21 g carbs, 17 g fat (3 g saturated fat), 90 mg cholesterol, 3 g fiber, 540 mg sodium

whole-wheat pita breads, 4

extra-virgin olive oil, 2 tsp plus 3 Tbsp

paprika, ¼ tsp

salt, ½ tsp

fresh lemon juice, 3 Tbsp

freshly ground pepper, ⅛ tsp

red leaf lettuce, ½ head, torn into bite-sized pieces

cooked skinless chicken or turkey breast, 3 cups (18 oz/560 g) shredded or cut into bite-sized pieces

English cucumber, 1 cup (5 oz/155 g) seeded and chopped

ripe tomato, 1 large, seeded and chopped

fresh flat-leaf parsley, 3 Tbsp chopped

red onion, 2 Tbsp chopped

MAKES 4 SERVINGS

1 Preheat oven to 375°F (190°C).

2 Using your fingers, separate each pita bread into 2 thin rounds. Brush outside of pita pieces lightly with 2 teaspoons olive oil total. Sprinkle lightly with paprika and ¼ teaspoon of salt. Arrange in a single layer, spiced side up, on 2 large baking sheets and bake until crisp, 10–12 minutes. Let cool. When cool enough to handle, break each round into 4 or 5 pieces.

3 In a large bowl, whisk together 3 tablespoons olive oil, lemon juice, remaining ¼ teaspoon salt, and pepper to make a dressing.

4 Add lettuce, chicken, cucumber, tomato, parsley, onion, and pita croutons to bowl and toss to mix and coat well. Serve right away.

This lemony, nutty pasta is delicious warm or cold, making it a great lunch-box option. Choose frozen or canned artichoke hearts for the pesto (the marinated ones will impart their own flavor) and be sure to drain thoroughly.

WHOLE-WHEAT ORZO WITH ARTICHOKE-ALMOND PESTO

almonds, ½ cup (2 oz/60 g)

dried whole-wheat orzo, 8 oz (250 g)

drained canned or thawed frozen artichoke hearts, 6

fresh flat-leaf parsley leaves, 1 cup packed (about 1 oz/30 g)

pitted green olives, ½ cup (2½ oz/75 g), chopped

olive oil, 3 Tbsp

finely grated lemon zest and juice, from 2 lemons

sea salt, ¼ tsp

freshly ground pepper, to taste

Parmesan cheese, 1 oz (30 g), shaved with a vegetable peeler (about ¼ cup)

MAKES 4 SERVINGS

1 Preheat oven to 350°F (180°C). Spread almonds on a baking sheet and toast in oven until lightly browned and fragrant, about 10 minutes. Immediately pour onto a plate to cool.

2 Meanwhile, bring a pot of lightly salted water to a boil. Add orzo and cook until tender but firm to the bite, about 8 minutes or according to package directions. Drain well.

3 While pasta is cooking, chop almonds, artichoke hearts, and parsley. Chop finely and uniformly, or coarsely for a more rustic, chunky texture. Transfer to a large serving bowl and add olives, olive oil, lemon zest and juice, salt, pepper, and cooked pasta. Stir to mix thoroughly. Gently fold in Parmesan and serve right away.

Look for whole-wheat orzo—a source of complex carbs—in the dried pasta section. Note that salting the cooking water increases the sodium content of the dish.

artichokes
- Extremely high in fiber
- Rich in magnesium, potassium, folate, and vitamin C
- Excellent source of antioxidants

fresh parsley
- Outstanding source of vitamin K, linked to bone health
- Has anti-inflammatory properties
- A natural breath freshener

per serving 460 calories, 16 g protein, 44 g carbs, 25 g fat (3.5 g saturated fat), 0 mg cholesterol, 9 g fiber, 550 mg sodium

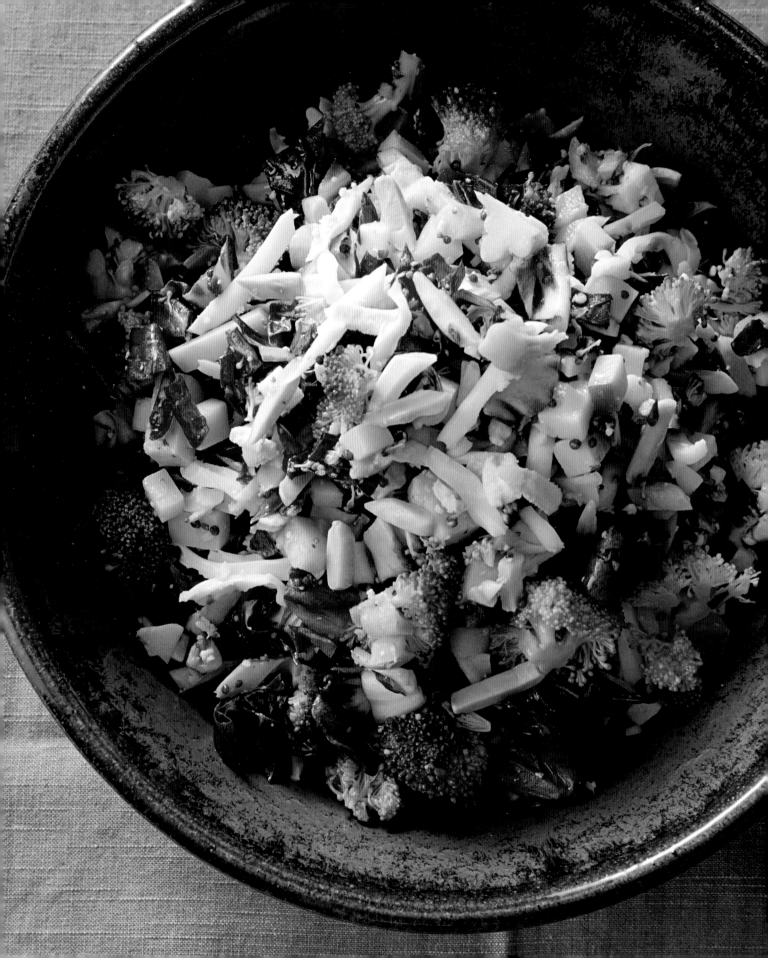

Whenever you make hard-boiled eggs, cook a few extra to have on hand for adding protein and heft to salads such as this one. If the flavor of raw broccoli is too strong for you, blanch the florets for a few minutes, then put them in ice water to halt the cooking.

CHOPPED SALAD WITH BROCCOLI, EGG & RADICCHIO

extra-virgin olive oil, ¼ cup (2 fl oz/60 ml)

fresh lemon juice, 3 Tbsp

whole-grain Dijon mustard, 1½ Tbsp

sea salt, ¼ tsp

broccoli, 1 lb (500 g), florets and tender stems, finely chopped

radicchio, 1 head (about 8 oz/250 g), cored and chopped

smoked or regular mozzarella cheese, 2 oz (60 g), cut into ¼-inch (6-mm) cubes

slivered or chopped almonds, ¼ cup (1½ oz/45 g)

hard-boiled eggs, 2, peeled and grated or finely chopped

MAKES 4 SERVINGS

1 In a large salad bowl, whisk together olive oil, lemon juice, mustard, and salt.

2 Add broccoli, radicchio, cheese, and almonds to bowl and stir gently to mix well and coat all ingredients with dressing. Add eggs and fold in gently just until combined. Serve right away.

There's plenty of protein packed into this hearty salad. For a lower-fat version, omit the cheese and remove the yolks from the hard-boiled eggs.

eggs
- Source of high-quality protein
- Linked to eye health
- A top source of choline, needed for brain health

almonds
- Rich in monounsaturated and polyunsaturated fats, potassium, and vitamin E
- Nuts are a good source of vegetarian protein
- Contain compounds shown to lower cholesterol

per serving 300 calories, 13 g protein, 12 g carbs, 25 g fat (4.5 g saturated fat), 100 mg cholesterol, 2 g fiber, 370 mg sodium

This modern take on a bread salad combines chewy cubes of whole-wheat sourdough with a tasty mixture of marinated tomatoes, tuna, and chickpeas. Use this recipe as a template for easy summer lunches, mixing different salad ingredients with the same dressing and bread.

PANZANELLA SALAD WITH TOMATOES, CHICKPEAS & TUNA

If you're watching your carb intake, you can omit the bread and you'll still have a delicious lunch salad, perfect for packing in a to-go container.

albacore tuna
- Contains heart-healthy omega-3 fatty acids
- Rich in potassium, iron, and selenium
- Instant source of lean protein

chickpeas
- Source of antioxidants linked to heart health
- High in fiber and protein
- Thought to help with blood-sugar regulation

per serving 440 calories, 24 g protein, 50 g carbs, 17 g fat (2.5 g saturated fat), 20 mg cholesterol, 13 g fiber, 650 mg sodium

crusty whole-wheat sourdough bread, 3 cups (6 oz/185 g) 1-inch (2.5-cm) cubes

extra-virgin olive oil, 4 Tbsp (2 fl oz/60 ml)

sherry vinegar or red wine vinegar, 3 Tbsp

low-sodium chickpeas, 1 can (15 oz/470 g), drained and rinsed

albacore tuna, 1 can (5 oz/155 g), water-packed, drained

English cucumber, 1 cup (5 oz/155 g) seeded and diced

radishes, ½ cup (2 oz/60 g) thinly sliced

red onion, ½, chopped

sea salt, ¼ tsp

freshly ground pepper, to taste

ripe tomatoes, 2 lb (1 kg), any color or variety

fresh basil leaves, from about ½ bunch, chopped

MAKES 4 SERVINGS

1 Preheat oven to 375°F (190°C). Place bread cubes on a baking sheet and toss with 1 tablespoon olive oil. Toast in oven until crisp and lightly browned on edges, about 15 minutes. Remove from oven and set aside.

2 While bread cubes are toasting, in a large salad bowl, whisk together vinegar and remaining 3 tablespoons olive oil. Add chickpeas, tuna, cucumber, radishes, onion, salt, and pepper. Stir to combine, using a fork to break up the tuna, and set aside.

3 If using large tomatoes, cut in half horizontally and gently squeeze out seeds, using your fingertip to nudge them if necessary. Cut into 1-inch (2.5-cm) chunks. Halve cherry tomatoes, if using. Add to bowl.

4 Just before serving, add bread cubes and stir to mix and coat well. Add basil and toss briefly to mix. Serve right away or let stand at room temperature for 15 minutes to allow flavors to blend.

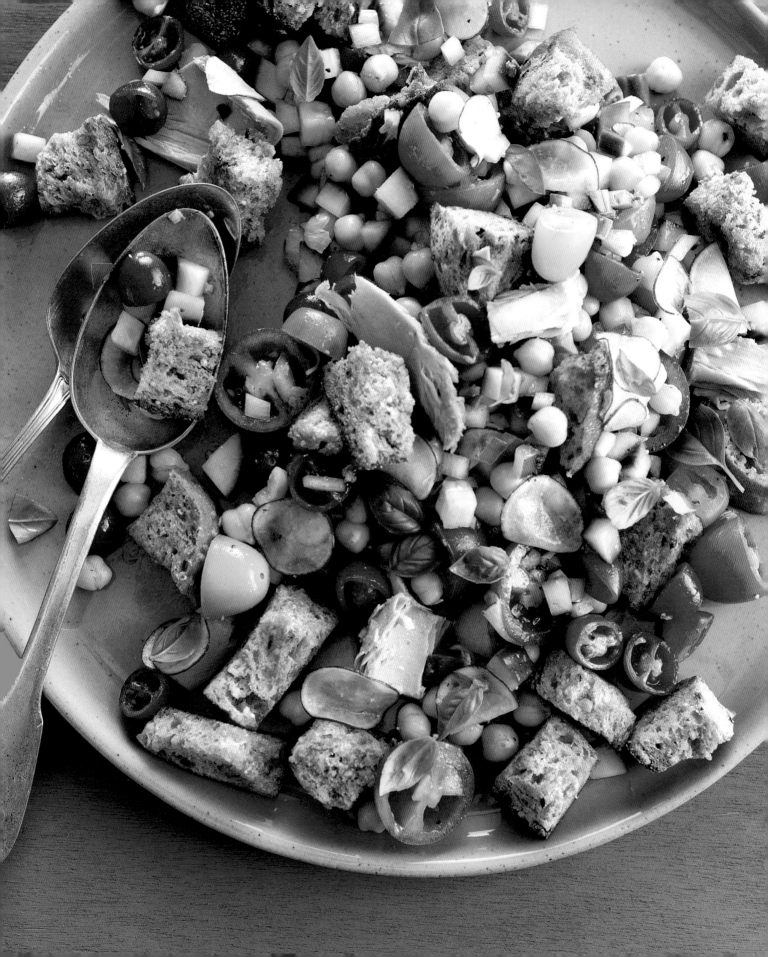

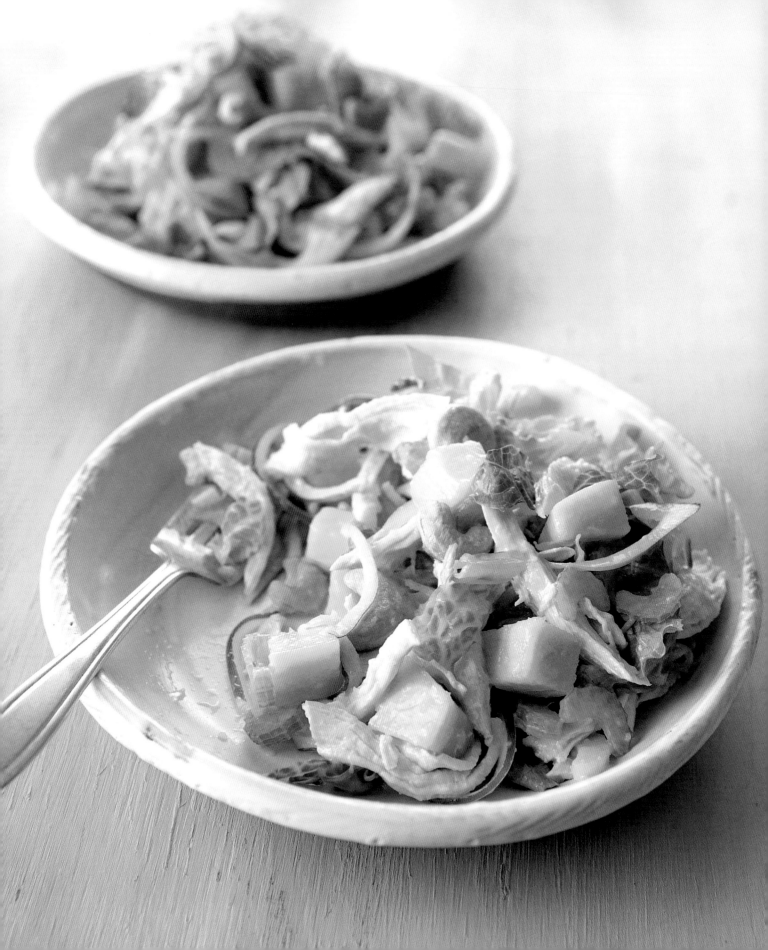

This bright, tangy salad is a smart way to make a meal of a purchased rotisserie chicken or poached chicken breast (page 81). The mango chutney adds depth of flavor to the dressing, but if you can't find it, sweeten the dressing to taste with honey.

CHICKEN & MANGO SALAD WITH CASHEWS

red onion, ½

ripe mangoes, 2

cooked skinless chicken breast, 3 cups (18 oz/560 g) shredded

celery, 2 stalks, thinly sliced

romaine lettuce, 4 cups (4 oz/125 g) sliced crosswise

grapeseed or peanut oil, ¼ cup (2 fl oz/60 ml)

champagne vinegar, 3 Tbsp

Dijon mustard, 1 Tbsp

garlic, 2 large cloves, pressed or minced

mango chutney, ½ cup (3 oz/90 g)

roasted cashews, ¼ cup (1½ oz/45 g)

MAKES 4 SERVINGS

1 Cut onion half crosswise into thin slices. Put onion slices in a colander and rinse well under cold running water. Drain thoroughly and set aside.

2 Working with 1 at a time, hold a mango upright on a cutting board. Using a sharp chef's knife, make downward cuts along each flat side of pit to separate from flesh. Remove skin with a vegetable peeler and cut flesh into 1-inch (2.5-cm) chunks. Put onion and mangoes in a large bowl and add chicken, celery, and lettuce.

3 In a bowl, whisk together oil, vinegar, mustard, garlic, and chutney until smooth to make a dressing.

4 Pour dressing over salad and toss gently to mix and coat well. Garnish with cashews and serve right away. Or, chill the salad and dressing separately for up to 4 hours and toss together right before serving, garnished with nuts.

You can omit the chicken for a delicious meatless salad; add a few more cashews for extra protein, if you like.

romaine lettuce
- Dark green color makes it nutritionally superior to paler lettuces
- Excellent source of folate and vitamins A and K
- Contains nutrients that support eye health

grapeseed oil
- Good source of vitamin E
- Good oil choice for high-heat cooking
- Light, neutral taste

per serving 490 calories, 36 g protein, 37 g carbs, 22 g fat (4.5 g saturated fat), 90 mg cholesterol, 4 g fiber, 270 mg sodium

A mildly spicy marinade brightened by fresh lime juice doubles as the dressing for this flavorful salad. As an even shorter cut to marinating and searing the tofu, you can substitute baked seasoned tofu, which can be found in most well-stocked grocery stores.

TOFU & WATERCRESS SALAD

Tofu is a smart choice for adding lean protein to your diet, even if you are a meat eater. Here, it adds heft to a salad of peppery greens and sweet bell pepper.

tofu
- Rich in heart-healthy nutrients
- Source of complete protein
- Contains the omega-3 fat alpha linolenic acid

watercress
- High in vitamin K, which helps with blood clotting
- Source of vitamins A and C
- A cruciferous vegetable, such as broccoli

per serving 200 calories, 9 g protein, 10 g carbs, 15 g fat (2 g saturated fat), 0 mg cholesterol, 2 g fiber, 95 mg sodium

rice vinegar, 3 Tbsp

fresh lime juice, 3 Tbsp

canola oil, 2 Tbsp

light brown sugar, 1 Tbsp firmly packed

low-sodium soy sauce, 1½ tsp

red pepper flakes, ¼ tsp

firm tofu, preferably nigari-style, 8 oz (250 g), sliced and cut into strips

watercress, torn into bite-sized pieces, or baby arugula leaves, 6 oz (185 g)

red bell pepper, 1, seeded and thinly sliced

roasted peanuts, ⅓ cup (2 oz/60 g), chopped

MAKES 4 SERVINGS

1 In a large bowl, whisk together vinegar, lime juice, and 1 tablespoon of oil. Add brown sugar, soy sauce, and red pepper flakes and whisk until sugar is dissolved. Add tofu and turn to coat well. Let stand for 15 minutes.

2 Heat remaining 1 tablespoon oil in a nonstick frying pan over medium heat. Using a slotted spoon, lift tofu out of marinade, letting liquid fall back into bowl, and add tofu to hot pan; reserve marinade in bowl. Cook, stirring often, until lightly browned, about 5 minutes. Remove from heat.

3 Add watercress and bell pepper to remaining marinade in bowl. Toss well to coat. Divide among 4 salad plates. Top each salad with tofu and peanuts and serve right away.

Turkey and cranberries is such a delightful pairing, it shouldn't be relegated to once-a-year at Thanksgiving. This versatile chutney is also delicious on crostini or crackers, and will keep, tightly sealed, for up to a week in the refrigerator.

TURKEY-SPINACH WRAPS WITH CRANBERRY CHUTNEY

dried cranberries, 1 cup (4 oz/125 g)

balsamic vinegar, 2 Tbsp

brown sugar, 2 Tbsp firmly packed

shallot, 1, chopped

finely grated orange zest, 1 tsp

salt, a pinch

freshly ground pepper

whole-wheat tortillas, 2 large

whipped light cream cheese, 4 Tbsp (1 oz/30 g)

roasted turkey breast, 4 oz (125 g), thinly sliced

baby spinach leaves, 2 big handfuls

MAKES 2 WRAPS

1 In a small saucepan, combine cranberries, vinegar, brown sugar, shallot, orange zest, salt, a few grindings of pepper, and ½ cup (4 fl oz/125 ml) water. Bring to a boil over high heat, then reduce heat to medium-low, cover, and simmer until cranberries are soft, about 5 minutes. Remove from heat and let cool. Transfer to a food processor and whirl until evenly combined and smooth.

2 Place 1 tortilla on a work surface on a sheet of waxed paper. Spread 2 tablespoons of cream cheese in a thin, even layer over entire surface of tortilla. Spread about 1 tablespoon of chutney evenly over cream cheese. Arrange half of turkey evenly over chutney, leaving a strip about 1 inch (2.5 cm) wide along one edge of tortilla uncovered. Arrange half of spinach evenly over turkey.

3 Roll up wrap, beginning at end opposite uncovered cream cheese and tucking tortilla snugly around ingredients. Press firmly on cream cheese end to seal. Turn seal side down and, using a serrated knife, cut wrap in half on diagonal. Repeat to assemble second wrap. Serve right away or wrap tightly in waxed paper, plastic wrap, or aluminum foil and take to go.

An antioxidant-packed cranberry chutney boosts the flavor of this lean lunch wrap, while spinach adds crunch and a wealth of nutrients.

turkey breast

- Source of lean protein, with fewer calories per serving than skinless chicken breast
- If buying roasted sliced turkey breast, choose a low-fat, low-sodium brand

dried cranberries

- Source of antioxidants that help reduce inflammation and cancer risk
- Known to have antibacterial properties

per wrap 510 calories, 18 g protein, 93 g carbs, 7 g fat (3.5 g saturated fat), 40 mg cholesterol, 7 g fiber, 910 mg sodium

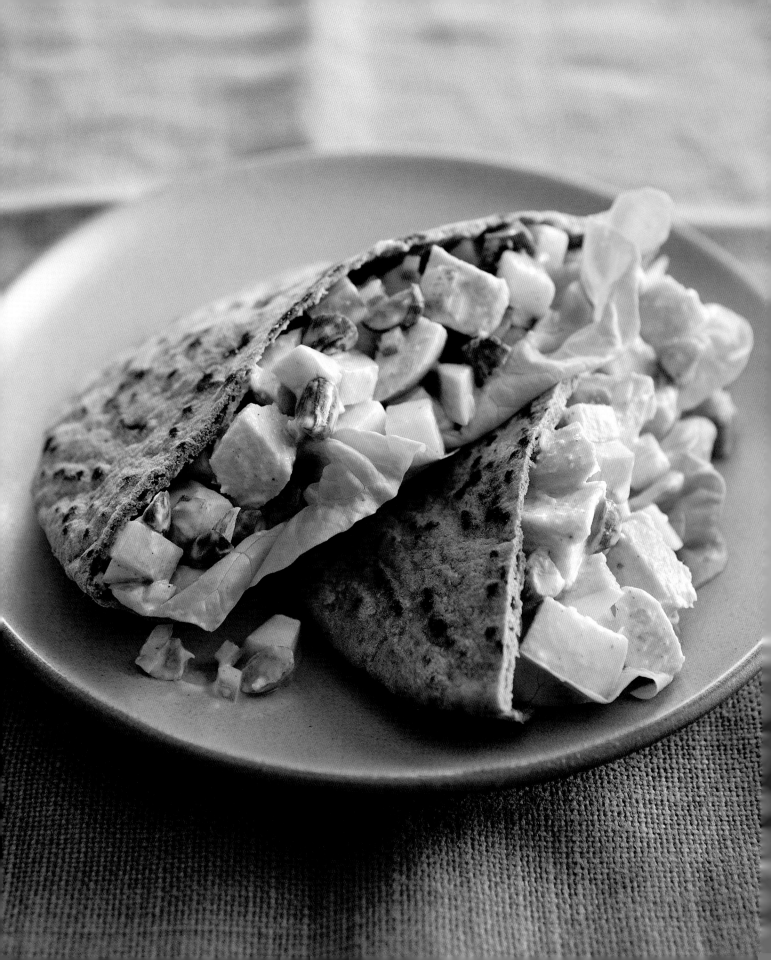

This tasty salad is great for picnics and lunch boxes. Keep it in mind when you're making chicken for dinner, and plan for leftovers. Or, drizzle 2 boneless, skinless chicken breasts with olive oil and lemon juice and bake in a 375°F (190°C) oven for about 30 minutes.

CURRIED CHICKEN–APPLE PITAS

almonds, ¼ cup (1¼ oz/37 g)

plain low-fat yogurt, 6 Tbsp (3 oz/90 g)

fresh lime juice, 2 Tbsp

honey, 1½ tsp

curry powder, 1 tsp

sea salt, ½ tsp

cooked skinless chicken breast, 1½ cups (9 oz/280 g) cubed or shredded

tart apple such as Granny Smith, 1, cored but not peeled, cut into small cubes

red onion, ¼ cup (1½ oz/45 g) minced

whole-wheat pita breads, 2, halved crosswise

butter lettuce leaves, 4

MAKES 2 SERVINGS

1 Preheat oven to 350°F (180°C). Spread almonds on a baking sheet and toast in oven until lightly browned and fragrant, about 10 minutes. Immediately pour onto a plate to cool, then chop coarsely and set aside.

2 In a large bowl, whisk together yogurt, lime juice, honey, curry powder, and salt. Add chicken, apple, onion, and almonds and stir to mix and coat well.

3 Using your fingers, gently open pita bread halves and tuck a lettuce leaf into each. Spoon chicken mixture into pockets, dividing evenly. Serve right away, or wrap well and pack to go.

Chicken salad is often loaded with mayonnaise, but not this version, which uses low-fat yogurt and wholesome flavorings, like lime juice, honey, and curry powder.

apples
- Rich in antioxidants shown to help regulate blood sugar
- Shown to aid in weight management
- Many active compounds are found in the skin

curry powder
- Rich in turmeric, a potent anti-inflammatory
- Contains compounds that may prevent cancer

per serving 530 calories, 45 g protein, 56 g carbs, 15 g fat (2.5 g saturated fat), 90 mg cholesterol, 9 g fiber, 910 mg sodium

This colorful sandwich, inspired by a Mexican torta, is packed full of fresh vegetables. You can use good-quality canned refried beans or make your own (page 177). If your market doesn't carry Mexican cheeses, crumbled fresh goat cheese is a good substitute.

AVOCADO & BLACK BEAN TORTAS

Black beans may seem like an unusual sandwich spread, but they add protein and flavor to this meatless meal. To reduce the fat, omit the cheese and cut the avocado in half.

black beans
- Excellent source of fiber
- A protein source that's inexpensive, nearly fat-free, and suitable for vegetarians
- Linked to heart health and blood-sugar regulation

cabbage
- Strongly linked to cancer prevention
- Excellent source of vitamin C

per sandwich 420 calories,
13 g protein, 44 g carbs,
23 g fat (6 g saturated fat),
20 mg cholesterol, 13 g fiber,
630 mg sodium

cabbage, 1 cup (3 oz/90 g) thinly shredded

ripe tomato, 1, seeded and chopped

radishes, 2 large, thinly sliced

fresh lime juice, 1 Tbsp

hot-pepper sauce, 1 tsp

crusty sandwich rolls, 2, split

low-sodium refried black beans, ⅔ cup (5 oz/155 g), warmed or at room temperature

***queso fresco* or *cotija* cheese**, ¼ cup (1½ oz/45 g) crumbled

ripe avocado, 1 small, pitted, peeled, and sliced

MAKES 2 SANDWICHES

1 Put cabbage, tomato, and radishes in a bowl and drizzle with lime juice and hot sauce and mix well. Set aside.

2 Using your fingers, remove some soft bread from insides of roll halves, making a hollow for sandwich filling. Toast rolls in a toaster or warm oven.

3 Spread half of refried beans over bottom half of each roll. Top with cheese and avocado slices. Divide vegetable mixture equally between sandwiches, mounding it on top of avocado. Replace top half of rolls and serve right away, or wrap well and pack to go.

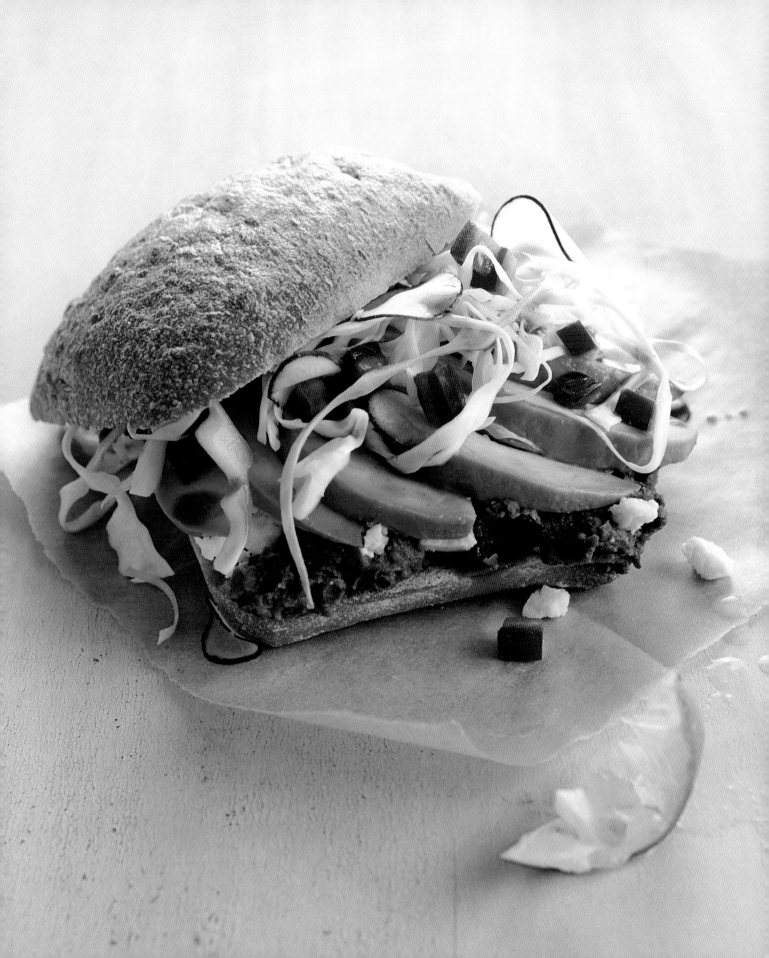

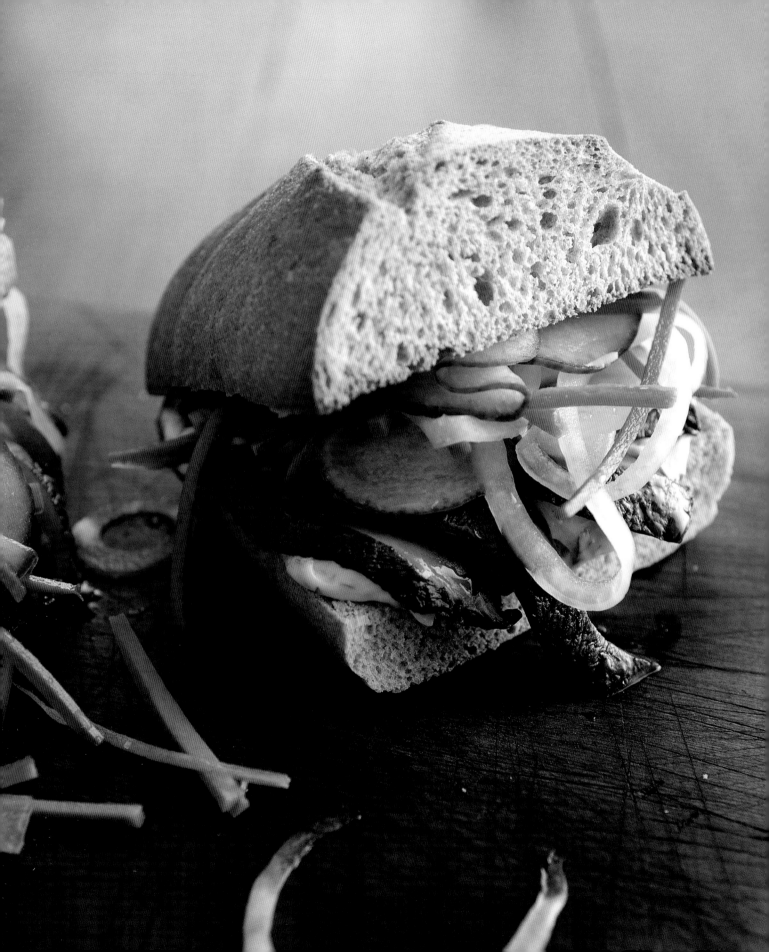

This hearty vegetarian sandwich hints at the flavors of a Vietnamese *bahn mi.* The vegetables get a quick vinegar bath as the mushroom caps roast. For a little spice, add some fresh jalapeño chile slices to the pickled vegetable mixture.

PORTOBELLO MUSHROOM SANDWICHES WITH PICKLED VEGETABLES

carrot, 1, peeled and cut into thin matchsticks

English cucumber, ¼ cup (1¼ oz/37 g) thinly sliced

sweet onion such as Vidalia or Walla Walla, 4 thin slices

rice vinegar, ¼ cup (2 fl oz/60 ml)

low-sodium soy sauce, 2 Tbsp

olive oil, 1 Tbsp

portobello mushroom caps, 2 large (about 4 inches/10 cm in diameter)

canola-oil mayonnaise, 2 Tbsp

fresh cilantro, 2 Tbsp minced

crusty whole-grain rolls, 2, split and toasted

MAKES 2 SANDWICHES

1 Preheat oven to 400°F (200°C).

2 Put carrot, cucumber, and onion slices in a bowl. Add vinegar and stir to mix and coat well. Set aside.

3 In a small bowl, stir together soy sauce and olive oil. Brush mushroom caps with soy-sauce mixture on all sides. Arrange on a baking sheet and roast until tender, 12–15 minutes. Remove from oven and let cool slightly. Using a serrated knife, slice mushrooms on diagonal into thin slices.

4 In another small bowl, stir together mayonnaise, cilantro, and ½ teaspoon rice vinegar from carrot and onion mixture. Spread bottom half of each roll with mayonnaise mixture and top with mushroom slices. Drain pickled vegetables and mound over mushroom slices, then add roll tops. Serve right away.

Juicy mushrooms are a low-fat yet satisfying stand-in for meat. To curb the sodium and carbs, use half the bread and make these open-faced sandwiches.

portobello mushrooms
- Excellent source of potassium
- Packed with niacin, a B vitamin that promotes heart health
- Contain compounds that fight inflammation and boost immunity

per sandwich 410 calories,
11 g protein, 59 g carbs,
16 g fat (2.5 g saturated fat),
0 mg cholesterol, 10 g fiber,
1120 mg sodium

Leftover cooked quinoa (page 81) works wonderfully in these savory, flavorful vegetarian burgers, which are enlivened with a hint of tangy barbecue sauce and pan-fried. Add even more toppings, if you like, such as baby spinach leaves, avocado, and tomato slices.

QUINOA—BLACK BEAN BURGERS

If you need a break from the standard frozen veggie burgers, or are looking for new ways to add protein to your diet, look no further than these simple, satisfying patties.

quinoa
- Provides complete protein
- Loaded with minerals such as iron, potassium, and magnesium
- Gluten-free

cumin
- May boost immune health and enhance digestion
- Rich source of iron

per serving 410 calories, 15 g protein, 63 g carbs, 12 g fat (2 g saturated fat), 45 mg cholesterol, 11 g fiber, 740 mg sodium

red onion, 1, ½ coarsely chopped, ½ sliced

garlic, 1 clove, coarsely chopped

low-sodium black beans, 1 can (15 oz/470 g), drained and rinsed

cooked quinoa, ½ cup (2½ oz/75 g)

fresh whole-wheat bread crumbs, ½ cup (2 oz/60 g)

large egg yolk, 1, lightly beaten

barbecue sauce, 2 Tbsp

ground cumin, 2 tsp

sea salt, ½ tsp

canola oil, 2 Tbsp

whole-wheat burger buns, 4, split and toasted

low-sodium ketchup or barbecue sauce, 4 Tbsp (2 oz/60 g)

MAKES 4 SERVINGS

1 In a food processor, whirl chopped onion and garlic until finely minced. Add black beans and pulse until mixture is a chunky purée. Transfer to a bowl.

2 Add quinoa, bread crumbs, egg yolk, barbecue sauce, cumin, and salt to bowl and fold in just until combined. Do not overmix. If you have time to chill mixture for about half an hour (or up to 1 day), the patties will be easier to form.

3 Using slightly moistened hands, shape bean mixture into 4 patties. Heat oil in a large nonstick frying pan over medium heat. Add patties and cook, carefully turning once, until browned, about 5 minutes per side. Spread cut sides of bun tops with ketchup. Place burgers on bun bottoms and top with onion slices. Serve right away.

There is a little assembly required here, but it takes just minutes and the results are crisp tortilla sandwiches with gooey melted cheese. You can substitute mango or pineapple for the papaya in the salsa. Serve with Baked Corn Chips (page 65) for scooping up extra salsa.

PINTO BEAN QUESADILLAS WITH PAPAYA SALSA

Mexican papaya, 3 cups (18 oz/560 g) seeded and diced

jicama, ½ cup (2½ oz/75 g) peeled and diced

red onion, 2 Tbsp minced

red Fresno chile, 1, seeded and minced

fresh cilantro, ¼ cup (⅓ oz/10 g) chopped

fresh lime juice, 3 Tbsp

sea salt, ¼ tsp

whole-wheat tortillas, 2 (8 inches/20 cm in diameter)

olive oil, 1 tsp

Monterey jack cheese, ½ cup (2 oz/60 g) shredded

low-sodium canned pinto beans, ½ cup (3½ oz/105 g) drained and rinsed

MAKES 2 SERVINGS

1 In a large bowl, combine papaya, jicama, onion, chile, cilantro, lime juice, and salt. Stir gently to mix well. Cover and refrigerate until ready to serve.

2 Brush tortillas lightly on one side with ½ teaspoon of olive oil total. Flip over and lay tortillas, oiled side down, on a work surface. Sprinkle half of each tortilla with one-fourth of cheese. Top each with half of beans, then remaining cheese. Fold each tortilla over into a half-moon and press gently to hold ingredients together.

3 Heat remaining ½ teaspoon olive oil in a nonstick frying pan over medium heat. Place 1 quesadilla in pan and cook until tortilla is lightly browned, about 2 minutes. Using a wide spatula, turn gently and cook until lightly browned on second side, about 2 minutes longer. Transfer to a plate and keep warm while you cook second quesadilla. Cut each quesadilla into 3 or 4 wedges. Serve right away with salsa. Store any unused salsa in an airtight container in the refrigerator for up to 2 days.

Quesadillas are a little less guilty when you add some heart-healthy beans and a nutritious tropical salsa.

pinto beans
- Good source of fiber and vegetarian protein
- Low in fat
- Linked to heart health and blood-sugar regulation

papayas
- Contain lycopene, believed to prevent certain cancers
- Rich in vitamins A and C
- Good source of folate for heart health

per serving 430 calories, 16 g protein, 59 g carbs, 15 g fat (7 g saturated fat), 25 mg cholesterol, 12 g fiber, 780 mg sodium

A special evening meal is the perfect way to unwind after a busy day. Decide how light—or hearty—to make yours depending on how much you've eaten throughout the day.

DINNER

QUICK-FIX IDEAS FOR DINNER

COOK IT IN A FLASH

VEGETARIAN BURRITOS Warm a splash of olive oil in a frying pan over medium heat. Add any chopped vegetables you have on hand, such as bell peppers, carrots, broccoli, or mushrooms. Sprinkle with a pinch of cumin and sauté until the vegetables are softened. Add 1 can (15 oz/470 g) low-sodium black beans, rinsed and drained, and a few dashes of hot sauce. Let the mixture cook, stirring occasionally, until the beans are warmed through. Season lightly with salt and pepper. Spoon over warmed whole-wheat tortillas and top with chopped fresh cilantro.

PEANUT TOFU STIR-FRY Combine equal parts light coconut milk, peanut butter, and lime juice in a bowl. Add a pinch of red pepper flakes. In a nonstick frying pan over medium-high heat, warm a splash of olive oil. Add cubed firm tofu, minced garlic, minced fresh ginger, and fresh or frozen peas and stir-fry until the tofu is browned and the peas are warmed through, about 5 minutes. Add the peanut sauce and stir-fry until thickened. Season lightly with salt or low-sodium soy sauce. Serve over cooked brown rice.

NO COOKING NEEDED

QUICK SALMON SALAD Combine mixed baby greens, sliced fennel or blanched green beans, halved cherry tomatoes, cooked white beans, and flaked salmon, poached or canned, in a large bowl. Toss with white wine vinegar and extra-virgin olive oil. Sprinkle with salt and pepper.

SPINACH COBB SALAD Toss together baby spinach leaves, sliced cooked beets, cubed avocado, shredded hard-cooked egg, and chopped smoked tofu or chopped cooked turkey breast in a large bowl. Toss with basic vinaigrette (page 215) or purchased honey-mustard vinaigrette.

MEZZE PLATE Create a combination plate filled with your favorite Mediterranean ingredients, like whole-wheat pita, Roasted Red Pepper Hummus (page 69), marinated artichokes, olives, purchased stuffed grape leaves (dolmas), and sliced tomatoes and cucumbers sprinkled with vinegar.

MAKE IT AHEAD

BASIL PESTO Combine 1 cup (1 oz/30 g) tightly
packed basil leaves; 1 clove garlic; ¼ cup
(2 fl oz/60 ml) olive oil; 2 tablespoons toasted
pine nuts; ¼ teaspoon salt; and several grindings
of pepper in a blender or food processor. Whirl
the ingredients until a coarse paste forms. Stir
in ⅓ cup (1½ oz/45 g) grated Parmesan cheese.
Store in an airtight container in the refrigerator
for up to 2 days or in the freezer for up to 3 months
(ice-cube trays work well for freezing). Toss
with cooked whole-wheat pasta, leftover poached
salmon or shredded cooked chicken, and halved
cherry tomatoes for a quick dinner.

POACHED SALMON Bring a large saucepan of
water to a boil over high heat. Add ½ teaspoon
salt, 1 thick yellow onion slice, 2 lemon slices, and
2 or 3 skinned salmon fillets. Reduce the heat until
the water is barely simmering and cook until the
salmon fillets are just opaque in the center, about
10 minutes per inch (2.5 cm) of thickness. Transfer
to a plate or cutting board to cool. Store in the
refrigerator for up to 2 days and flake or chop as
needed for salads, pastas, or sandwiches.

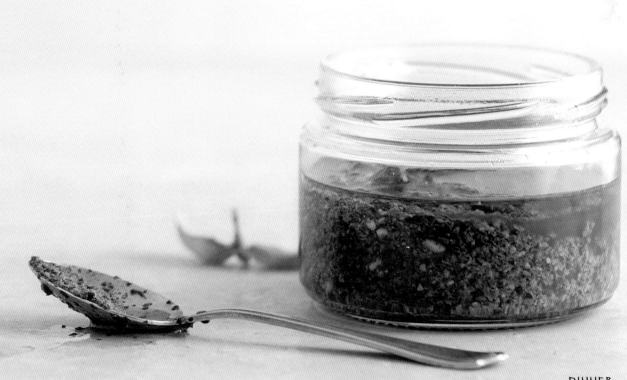

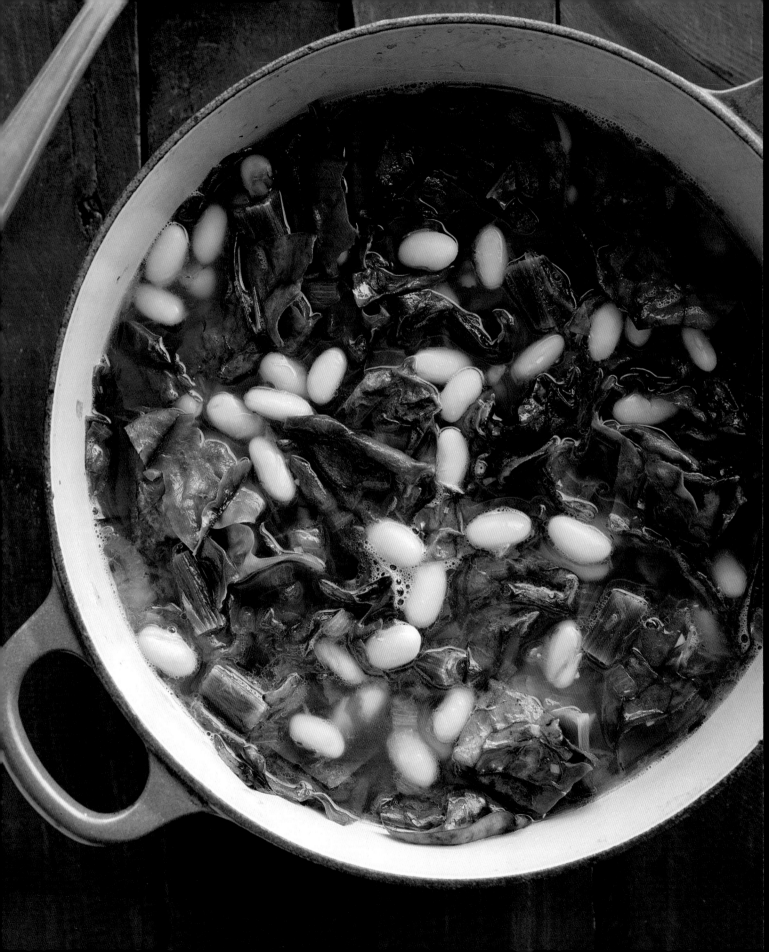

Taking a little extra time to cook sweet onions over low heat until tender and mellow adds a nice caramelized flavor to this simple soup, which you can assemble otherwise with little effort. For extra richness, add a Parmesan cheese rind to the broth as the soup simmers.

WHITE BEAN SOUP WITH RED CHARD

olive oil, 2 Tbsp

sweet onions such as Vidalia or Walla Walla, 2 large (about 1 lb/500 g total weight), finely chopped

red chard, 2 bunches (about 1 lb/500 g total weight), leaves torn into bite-sized pieces, ribs and stems chopped

sea salt, ⅛ tsp

garlic, 2 cloves, pressed or minced

dried thyme, ¼ tsp

low-sodium chicken or vegetable broth or stock, 6 cups (48 fl oz/1.5 l)

low-sodium cannellini or white kidney beans, 2 cans (15 oz/470 g each), drained and rinsed

Parmesan cheese, ¼ cup (1 oz/30 g) freshly grated

MAKES 6 SERVINGS

1 Heat olive oil in a large pot over medium-high heat. Add onions and chard ribs and stems and stir to coat well with oil. Sprinkle in salt, reduce heat to medium, and sauté until vegetables are softened, about 10 minutes.

2 Add garlic and thyme and cook, stirring constantly, until garlic is fragrant but not browned, 1–2 minutes longer.

3 Add broth and bring to a simmer. Add beans and chard leaves, return to a simmer, and cook, stirring occasionally, until chard is wilted, 5–7 minutes. Ladle soup into bowls and top each serving with Parmesan cheese. Serve right away.

This brothy soup is low in fat and loaded with nutritional heavy-hitters, including chard and white beans. If you're watching your sodium intake, omit the Parmesan cheese.

chard
- Rich in nutrients that promote bone and eye health
- Promotes detoxification
- Fights inflammation

sweet onions
- Good source of folate, vitamin B6, and vitamin C
- May help fight some kinds of cancer
- Rich in quercetin, a powerful antioxidant

per serving 200 calories, 12 g protein, 25 g carbs, 6 g fat (1.5 g saturated fat), 0 mg cholesterol, 5 g fiber, 840 mg sodium

On a cold night, there's nothing more satisfying than a hearty bowl of soup like this one, chock-full of bright vegetables and tender lentils. Unlike other dried legumes, lentils need no presoaking, so think of this recipe when you want homemade soup but are short on time.

VEGETABLE & LENTIL SOUP

Lentils add fiber and heft to this nourishing soup. Use vegetable broth, or all water, to make it a vegetarian dish.

spinach
- Good source of folate and carotenoids
- Rich in vitamins and minerals
- Linked to blood clotting and bone health

lentils
- Excellent source of fiber, which helps regulate blood sugar
- Extremely rich in heart-healthy nutrients like folate and potassium

per serving 490 calories, 31 g protein, 72 g carbs, 8 g fat (1 g saturated fat), 0 mg cholesterol, 33 g fiber, 910 mg sodium

brown lentils, 2 cups (14 oz/440 g)
olive oil, 2 Tbsp
yellow onion, 1, chopped
carrot, 1, peeled and chopped
garlic, 1 clove, pressed or minced
low-sodium chicken broth or stock, 4 cups (32 fl oz/1 l)
low-sodium diced or crushed tomatoes, 1 can (28 oz/875 g)

smoked paprika, 1 tsp
ground cumin, 1 tsp
salt, ½ tsp
freshly ground pepper, ¼ tsp
baby spinach, 4 oz (125 g)
dry sherry, 2 Tbsp

MAKES 4 SERVINGS

1 Pick over lentils for stones or grit. Rinse in a colander under cold running water and drain thoroughly.

2 Heat olive oil in a large pot over medium-high heat. Add onion and cook, stirring often, until softened, about 5 minutes. Add carrot and cook until carrot is softened, about 3 minutes longer. Add garlic and cook, stirring, until fragrant but not browned, about 30 seconds.

3 Stir in broth, 2 cups (16 fl oz/500 ml) water, lentils, tomatoes with their juices, paprika, cumin, salt, and pepper. Bring to a boil. Reduce heat to low, cover, and simmer gently until lentils are very tender, about 20 minutes. Chop spinach coarsely and stir into soup. Cook, uncovered, just until spinach is wilted, about 1 minute. Stir in sherry. Ladle soup into bowls and serve hot.

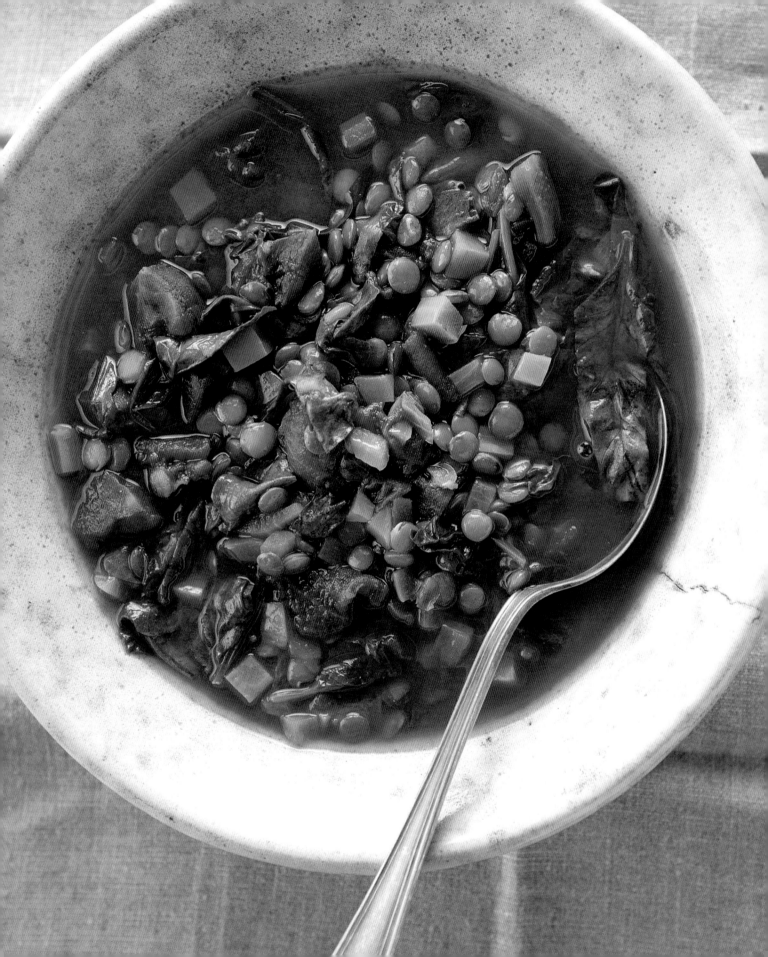

Soba noodles are typically made from buckwheat flour, although some are a blend of buckwheat and regular wheat; either will work well in this recipe. The key to cooking them is to boil them gently in plenty of water and then rinse them immediately under cold water.

SESAME SOBA NOODLES WITH BOK CHOY

Make pasta the Japanese way for an easy dish that's full of flavor and goodness. If you're on a gluten-free diet, make sure the noodles are made from 100 percent buckwheat.

buckwheat noodles
- Great way to add whole grains to your diet
- Good source of fiber, which contributes to heart health
- Source of complete protein and minerals like magnesium

sesame seeds
- Source of copper, an anti-inflammatory, and calcium
- Linked to reducing cholesterol and regulating blood pressure

per serving 350 calories,
9 g protein, 48 g carbs,
15 g fat (2 g saturated fat),
0 mg cholesterol, 2 g fiber,
670 mg sodium

dried soba noodles, 8 oz (250 g)

olive oil, 2 Tbsp

fresh ginger, 1 Tbsp minced or grated

garlic, 1 clove, pressed or minced

baby bok choy, 1 lb (500 g), trimmed and cut into 1-inch (2.5-cm) pieces

toasted sesame oil, 2 Tbsp

low-sodium soy sauce, 1 Tbsp

fresh lemon juice, 2 tsp

toasted sesame seeds, 1 Tbsp

MAKES 4 SERVINGS

1 Bring a large pot of water to a boil over high heat. Add soba and cook gently, stirring once or twice, just until tender, about 7 minutes. Drain in a colander, reserving 3 tablespoons cooking water, and immediately place noodles under cold running water to cool and rinse well.

2 Heat olive oil in a large frying pan over medium heat. Add ginger and garlic and cook until fragrant, about 1 minute. Add bok choy and stir to coat thoroughly with oil. Add reserved pasta cooking water to pan. Cover and steam until bok choy is tender, about 2 minutes.

3 Place soba in pan with bok choy and add sesame oil, soy sauce, lemon juice, and sesame seeds. Stir to mix well and cook just until heated through, about 2 minutes. Serve right away.

The fish counter and freezer case at the supermarket can help you put together a quick seafood stew like this one, whose spicy flavor is a nod to quinoa's Peruvian roots. Ask for squid that's been cleaned and cut into rings and shrimp that's been peeled and deveined.

SPICY SEAFOOD STEW WITH QUINOA

quinoa, 1½ cups (12 oz/375 g)

olive oil, 1 Tbsp

yellow onion, 1, halved lengthwise and thinly sliced crosswise

garlic, 2 cloves, pressed or minced

low-sodium crushed tomatoes, 1 can (28 oz/875 g)

hot green chiles such as jalapeños, 1 or 2, seeded and minced

ground cumin, ½ tsp

chili powder, ½ tsp

salt, ¼ tsp

shrimp, 12 oz (375 g) large, peeled and deveined

tilapia or other firm white fish, 8 oz (250 g), cut into 1-inch (2.5-cm) chunks

squid rings, 4 oz (125 g), fresh or thawed frozen

fresh cilantro, 2 Tbsp chopped

MAKES 4 SERVINGS

1 In a saucepan, bring 2 cups (16 fl oz/500 ml) water to a boil over high heat. Put quinoa in a fine-mesh strainer and rinse under cold running water. Add quinoa to boiling water, stir once, and return to a boil. Reduce heat to medium-low, cover, and cook until water is absorbed and quinoa is tender, 18–20 minutes.

2 Meanwhile, heat olive oil in a large, deep-sided frying pan over medium-high heat. Add onion and garlic and cook, stirring often, until onion is soft and golden, 8–10 minutes. Add crushed tomatoes with their juices, 1¼ cups (10 fl oz/310 ml) water, chile(s), cumin, chili powder, and salt. Stir well and bring to a simmer.

3 Add shrimp, tilapia, and squid and fold gently to distribute. Reduce heat to maintain a gentle simmer. Cover pan and cook until shrimp and fish are opaque throughout (cut into one piece to test), 3–4 minutes. Stir in cilantro and remove from heat.

4 Spoon quinoa into shallow bowls. Ladle stew on top and serve hot.

This seafood stew, aromatic with exotic spices, is served over a bed of quinoa for a low-fat, protein-rich meal.

quinoa
- Excellent source of complex carbs for prolonged energy
- Gluten free
- Rich in minerals such as iron, potassium, and magnesium

squid
- Very lean source of protein
- Rich in selenium, a mineral that boosts immunity and protects against cancer
- Provides choline, a nutrient that enhances brain health and memory

per serving 460 calories, 38 g protein, 54 g carbs, 10 g fat (1.5 g saturated fat), 200 mg cholesterol, 7 g fiber, 700 mg sodium

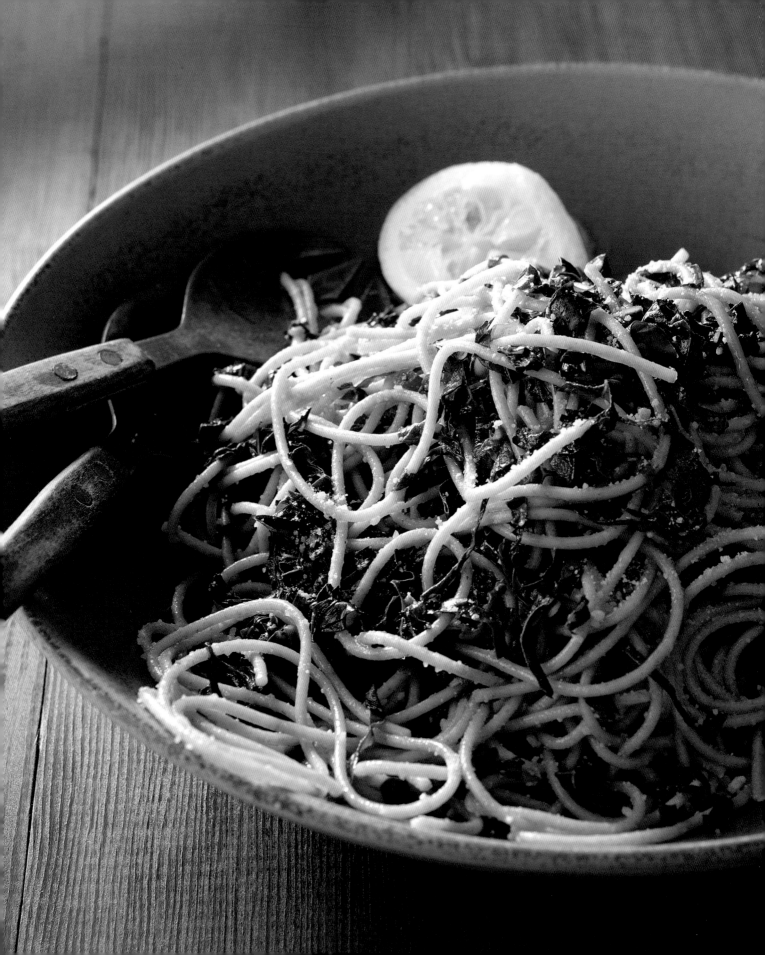

This tangle of noodles and garlic-laden ribbons of kale and chard is a delicious way to eat your greens. Dinosaur kale, also known as lacinato or Tuscan kale, has dark blueish-green leaves and a more delicate flavor than curly kale.

SPAGHETTI WITH GARLICKY GREENS

whole-wheat spaghetti or linguini, 12 oz (375 g)

red or green chard, 1 bunch (about ½ lb/250 g)

dinosaur (lacinato) kale, 1 bunch (about ½ lb/250 g)

olive oil, 4 Tbsp (2 fl oz/60 ml)

garlic, 4 cloves, pressed or minced

red pepper flakes, ¼ tsp

Parmesan cheese, ¼ cup (1 oz/30 g) freshly grated

sea salt, ¼ tsp

lemon wedges, for serving

MAKES 4 SERVINGS

1 Bring a large pot of lightly salted water to a boil. Add pasta and cook until just tender, about 9 minutes, or according to package directions.

2 Meanwhile, rinse greens and tear leaves from their tough ribs and stems, discarding ribs and stems. Stack leaves and fold or roll up and slice them thinly. Transfer greens to a colander and rinse under cold running water, then drain well.

3 Heat 2 tablespoons of olive oil in a large frying pan over medium-high heat. Add garlic and red pepper flakes and cook, stirring constantly, until garlic is fragrant but not browned, about 1 minute. Add greens and stir to coat evenly with oil. (If they don't all fit at once, add in handfuls after allowing first batch to wilt.) Cook, stirring occasionally, until greens are tender, about 5 minutes, adding a few tablespoons of pasta cooking water to pan if needed to prevent sticking.

4 Drain pasta and return to warm pot. Add cooked greens, Parmesan, salt, and remaining 2 tablespoons olive oil and stir to mix well. Divide evenly among pasta plates or bowls and serve right away. Pass lemon wedges at the table.

This recipe proves that pasta doesn't need to be a guilty indulgence. Note that salting the pasta cooking water will increase the sodium content of the dish.

whole-wheat pasta
- An easy way to add whole grains and fiber into your diet
- Slowly digested so it helps you stay full

garlic
- Rich in compounds linked to cancer prevention
- May lower cholesterol and blood pressure
- Has antimicrobial properties

per serving 490 calories, 18 g protein, 73 g carbs, 17 g fat (3 g saturated fat), 5 mg cholesterol, 2 g fiber, 400 mg sodium

This celebration of tomatoes is a nearly no-cook pasta dish, perfect for summer evenings when it's too hot to linger at the stove. Reserve this delicious pasta for when tomatoes are juicy and at their peak; the rest of the year, substitute tomato sauce (page 215).

FRESH TOMATO & BASIL PASTA

To lower the fat content, you can reduce or omit the mozzarella. Note that salting the pasta cooking water increases the sodium content of the dish.

tomatoes
- Good source of vitamins A and C, as well as other antioxidants
- High in lycopene, thought to protect against cancer
- Help prevent wrinkles and keep skin supple

fresh basil
- Contains volatile oils that fight inflammation
- Excellent source of vitamin K

per serving 450 calories, 18 g protein, 44 g carbs, 19 g fat (7 g saturated fat), 40 mg cholesterol, 7 g fiber, 460 mg sodium

extra-virgin olive oil, ¼ cup (2 fl oz/60 ml)

balsamic vinegar, 2 Tbsp

garlic, 1 clove, pressed or minced

sea salt, ½ tsp

freshly ground black pepper, to taste

ripe heirloom tomatoes, 3 lb (1.5 kg), cored

whole-wheat penne, 12 oz (375 g)

mozzarella *bocconcini*, 8 oz (250 g), halved

fresh basil leaves, 1 cup packed (1 oz/30 g), torn into pieces

Parmesan cheese, ¼ cup (1 oz/30 g) freshly grated

red pepper flakes (optional)

MAKES 6 SERVINGS

1 Bring a large pot of lightly salted water to a boil over high heat.

2 Meanwhile, in a large bowl, whisk together olive oil, vinegar, garlic, salt, and black pepper.

3 Cut tomatoes in half horizontally and gently squeeze out seeds and discard, using your fingertip to nudge them if necessary. Chop tomatoes into bite-sized chunks. Add to bowl and stir gently to coat. Set aside.

4 Add pasta to boiling water and cook until just tender, about 9 minutes, or according to package directions. Drain well.

5 Add warm pasta to bowl with tomato mixture and stir gently to coat well. Add *bocconcini* and basil and mix gently to distribute evenly and help cheese melt. Serve right away, passing Parmesan and red pepper flakes, if using, at the table.

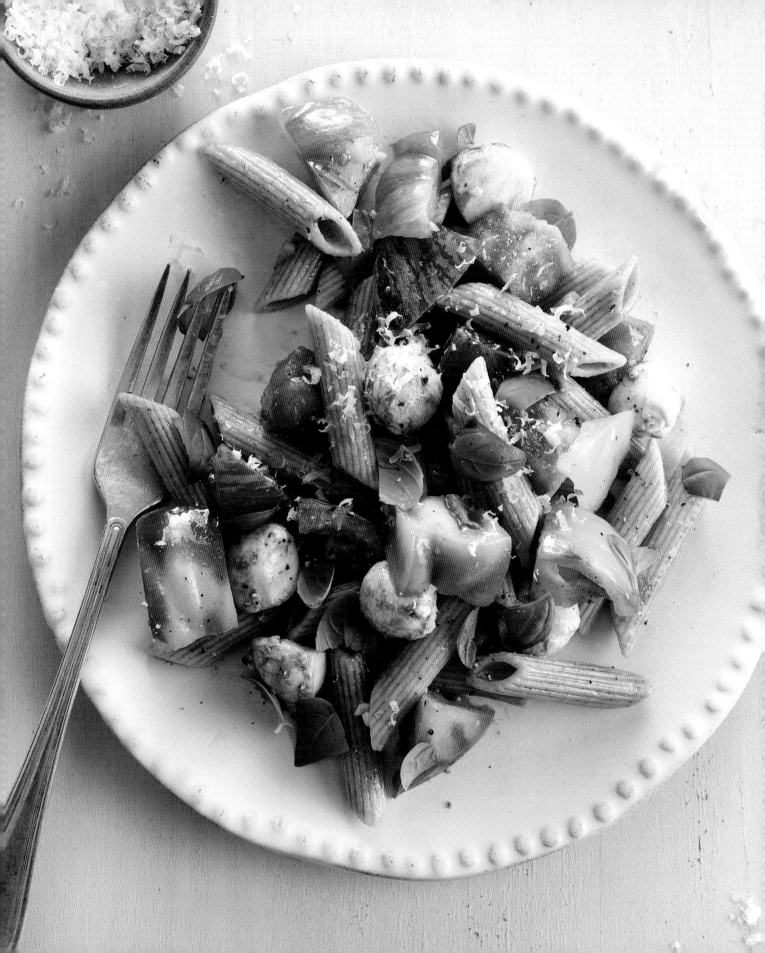

Farro is a nutty-tasting grain similar in texture to barley; choose semi-pearled rather than whole-grain *farro,* as it cooks much more quickly. You can buy preshaved Parmesan cheese, or shave your own easily from a wedge using a vegetable peeler.

FARRO WITH CHICKPEAS, PROSCIUTTO & CHARD

semi-pearled *farro*, 1 cup (7 oz/220 g)

red chard, 1 bunch (about ½ lb/250 g), tough stems removed

olive oil, 4 Tbsp (2 fl oz/60 ml)

prosciutto, 2 oz (60 g), chopped (about ½ cup)

fresh sage leaves, ¼ cup packed (⅓ oz/10 g)

low-sodium chickpeas, 1 can (15 oz/470 g), drained and rinsed

fresh lemon juice, 2 Tbsp

Parmesan cheese, ⅓ cup (1½ oz/45 g) shaved

freshly ground pepper, to taste

MAKES 4 SERVINGS

For a meatless meal that's also lower in sodium, omit the prosciutto. Note that adding salt to the cooking water increases the sodium content of the dish.

farro
- Richer in protein than most other grains
- Excellent source of complex carbs and fiber to promote fullness and satiety

chickpeas
- Source of antioxidants linked to heart health
- High in fiber and protein
- Thought to help with blood-sugar regulation

per serving 460 calories, 21 g protein, 59 g carbs, 23 g fat (4 g saturated fat), 15 mg cholesterol, 14 g fiber, 660 mg sodium

1 Bring a saucepan of lightly salted water to a boil. Add *farro* and simmer, stirring occasionally, until grains are tender, 18–20 minutes. Drain.

2 Meanwhile, trim stem ends of chard and cut crosswise into thin slivers. Place in a colander and rinse well.

3 Heat 1 tablespoon of olive oil in a frying pan over medium heat. Add prosciutto and sage leaves. Stir until prosciutto is beginning to brown and both prosciutto and sage are crisp, about 3 minutes. Remove from pan using tongs or a slotted spoon and place in a large bowl.

4 Raise heat to medium-high. Add 1 tablespoon of olive oil to pan and then add chard. Turn to coat with oil and cook, stirring often, until chard ribs are tender, about 5 minutes. Add 1–2 tablespoons water if pan becomes dry.

5 Add *farro*, chard, and chickpeas to prosciutto mixture. Stir in lemon juice and remaining 2 tablespoons olive oil. Mix well. Add Parmesan cheese and pepper and mix gently. Serve right away.

Frozen brown rice, available at many well-stocked supermarkets, steams or microwaves quickly and is a good shortcut for enjoying whole-grain rice with stir-fries like this one. Alternatively, make a double batch whenever you're cooking rice and freeze the leftovers.

SPRING STIR-FRY WITH PEAS & SHRIMP

slender asparagus, ¾ lb (375 g)

canola oil, 1 Tbsp

garlic, 2 cloves, pressed or minced

fresh ginger, 1-inch (2.5-cm) piece, peeled and grated or minced

shelled fresh peas, 1 cup (5 oz/155 g)

shrimp, ¾ lb (375 g) medium, peeled and deveined

low-sodium chicken or vegetable broth or stock, ⅓ cup (3 fl oz/80 ml)

low-sodium soy sauce, 1 Tbsp

cooked brown rice, 2 cups (10 oz/315 g)

MAKES 4 SERVINGS

1 Break off and discard tough stem ends from asparagus. Cut spears on diagonal into 1¼-inch (3-cm) lengths.

2 Heat oil in a wok or large frying pan over medium-high heat. Add garlic and ginger and cook, stirring constantly, until garlic is fragrant but not browned, about 30 seconds. Add asparagus and peas and stir to coat with oil. Cook for 1 minute.

3 Sprinkle 3 tablespoons water into pan. Cover and cook just until vegetables are bright green, 1–2 minutes. Add shrimp and cook, uncovered, stirring often, until opaque throughout, 2–3 minutes. Add broth and soy sauce and bring to a simmer, then immediately remove from heat.

4 Serve right away, with brown rice.

Stir-frying is a healthy, quick-cooking technique well suited for busy weeknights. Use any tender vegetables and lean proteins you have on hand.

asparagus
- Rich in antioxidants
- High in vitamins A and K
- Good source of vitamin C, folate, and potassium

brown rice
- Excellent source of slowly digested complex carbs
- Contains more than five times the fiber of white rice
- Packed with manganese, needed for a healthy metabolism

per serving 250 calories, 18 g protein, 34 g carbs, 5 g fat (.5 g saturated fat), 105 mg cholesterol, 6 g fiber, 670 mg sodium

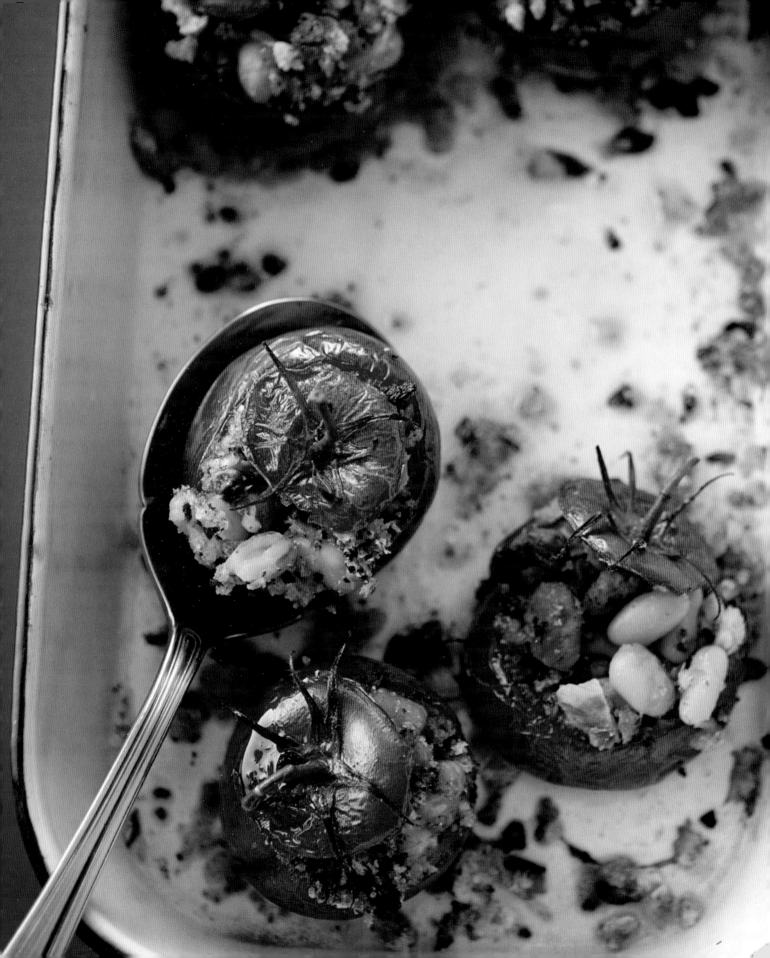

The beauty of this dish lies in its basic ingredients, most of which you probably already have in your pantry. For a striking presentation, reserve the tomato tops, with the stems attached, and place them over the filling before baking.

BAKED TOMATOES WITH TUNA, WHITE BEANS & BREAD CRUMBS

olive oil, 2 Tbsp

crusty artisan-style bread, 2 slices (about ½ inch/12 mm thick)

garlic, 1 clove, peeled but left whole

fresh flat-leaf parsley, 2 Tbsp chopped

ripe tomatoes, 4 large or 8 small

albacore tuna, 1 can (5 oz/155 g) water-packed, drained

low-sodium canned cannellini or butter beans, ½ cup (3½ oz/105 g), drained and rinsed

red onion, 2 Tbsp minced

capers, 1 Tbsp, drained

sherry vinegar, 1 tsp

MAKES 2 SERVINGS

1 Preheat oven to 300°F (150°C). Lightly grease a baking dish with 1 teaspoon of olive oil.

2 Place bread slices on a baking sheet and bake until crisp and beginning to brown, about 15 minutes. Scrape garlic clove on one side of each warm bread slice. Let bread cool, then tear into chunks and put in a food processor. Whirl to make uniform coarse crumbs. Transfer bread crumbs to a bowl and mix with 2 teaspoons of olive oil and 1 tablespoon of parsley. Raise oven temperature to 375°F (190°C).

3 Cut a uniform opening in top of each tomato around stem and remove tops. Using a melon baller, gently scoop out core and seeds of tomatoes, leaving side walls intact. Arrange tomatoes, cut side up, in prepared dish.

4 In a large bowl, combine tuna, beans, onion, capers, vinegar, remaining 1 tablespoon olive oil, and remaining 1 tablespoon parsley. Stir to mix, using a fork to break up tuna. Spoon filling into tomatoes, dividing it evenly and mounding it slightly on top. Cover filling generously with bread crumbs.

5 Bake until bread crumbs are golden and sides of tomatoes are soft and skins have just begun to split, 20–25 minutes. Let cool slightly and serve.

A hollowed-out tomato makes a perfect baking vessel; here, tuna, white beans, and bread crumbs form a hearty filling.

albacore tuna
- Contains heart-healthy omega-3 fatty acids
- Rich in potassium and selenium
- Instant source of lean protein

white beans
- Combination of slowly digested protein and fiber keeps you full
- Linked to heart health and cancer prevention
- Rich source of cholesterol-lowering soluble fiber

per serving 470 calories, 30 g protein, 59 g carbs, 18 g fat (2.5 g saturated fat), 30 mg cholesterol, 8 g fiber, 760 mg sodium

Oranges, scallops, and even onions are at their best in the wintertime, and these lively flavors will help brighten up a gloomy evening. Take care not to overcook scallops, as they go quickly from perfectly tender to tough and chewy.

SEARED SCALLOPS WITH ORANGES

If you think scallops are only for fancy affairs, think again: they are a versatile and quick-cooking protein. Serve them over a simple orange salad for a refreshing, low-calorie meal.

sea scallops
- Extremely lean source of protein
- Excellent source of vitamin B12, an important nutrient for heart health
- Good source of selenium, an antioxidant that may protect against cancer

per serving 190 calories, 15 g protein, 17 g carbs, 7 g fat (1 g saturated fat), 25 mg cholesterol, 3 g fiber, 660 mg sodium

red onion, ½, thinly sliced
rice vinegar, 4 tsp
oranges, 3
capers, 1 Tbsp drained and rinsed
extra-virgin olive oil, 2 Tbsp
sea scallops, 1 lb (500 g), 1½–2 inches (4–5 cm) in diameter

salt, ¼ tsp
freshly ground pepper, ¼ tsp, plus more to taste
fresh flat-leaf parsley or mint, 2 Tbsp chopped

MAKES 4 SERVINGS

1 Put onion slices in a colander and rinse well under cold running water. Drain thoroughly, then transfer to a small bowl and stir in rice vinegar. Set aside.

2 Remove 1 teaspoon finely grated zest from 1 orange; set zest aside. Using a sharp knife, cut a thin slice off both ends of each orange, then cut away peel and bitter white pith, following fruit's curve. Cut oranges in half lengthwise, then slice crosswise into thin half-moons. In a bowl, combine orange slices with reserved zest, capers, and 1 tablespoon of olive oil. Set aside.

3 Sprinkle scallops with salt and ¼ teaspoon pepper. Heat remaining 1 tablespoon olive oil in a large nonstick frying pan over medium-high heat. Add scallops and cook, turning once, until browned on both sides and opaque in center, 4–5 minutes total.

4 Add onion (with vinegar), parsley, and a few grindings of pepper to orange mixture and toss gently to combine. Divide orange salad among 4 dinner plates and top with warm scallops, dividing them evenly. Serve right away.

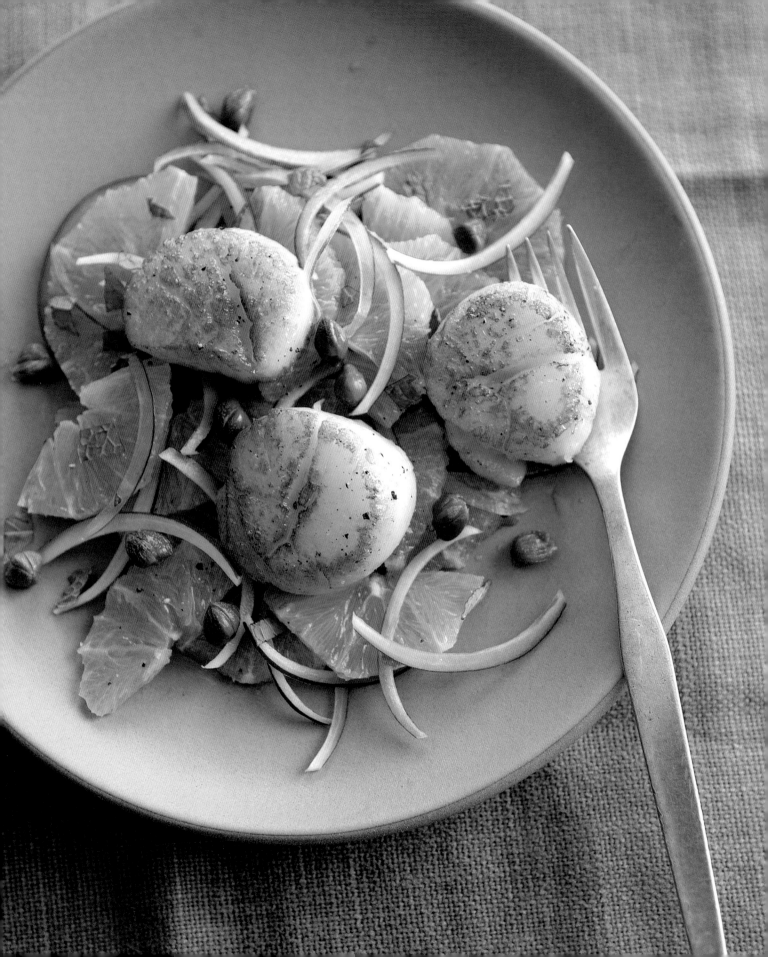

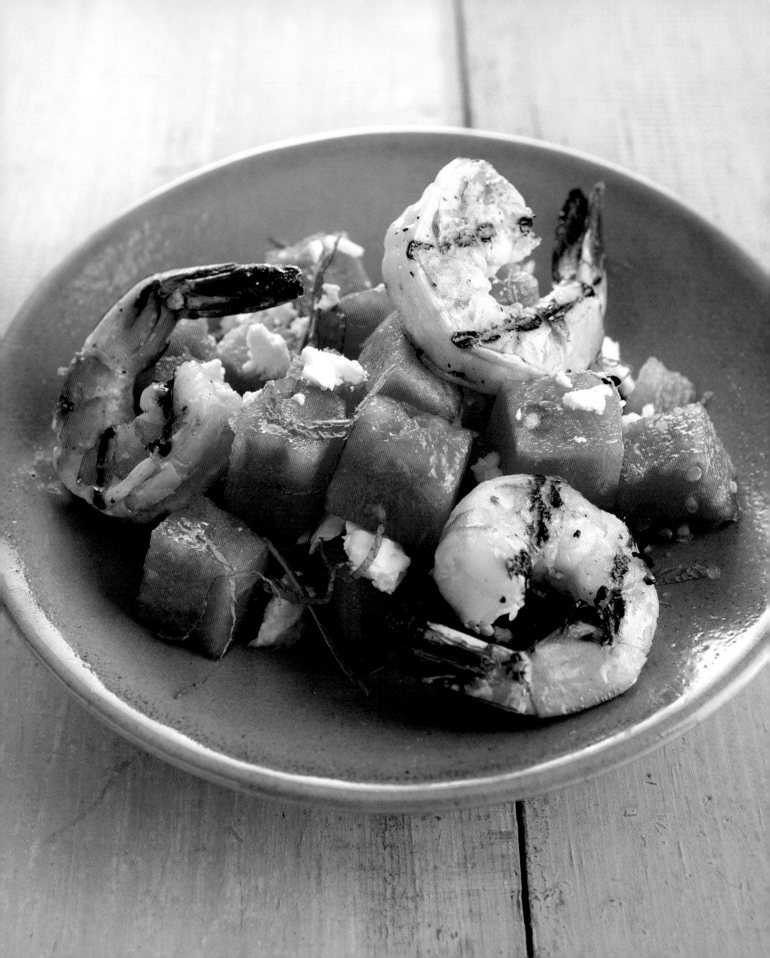

A minty watermelon salad paired with simple grilled shrimp makes a light and refreshing summer meal. The recipe is easy to double or triple to serve a crowd. To serve family-style, mound the watermelon salad on a platter and arrange the shrimp skewers on top.

GRILLED SHRIMP WITH WATERMELON & FETA

fresh orange juice, 3 Tbsp

fresh lime juice, 4 Tbsp (2 fl oz/60 ml)

salt, a pinch

seedless watermelon, 1 small, about 3 lb (1.5 kg)

fresh mint leaves, 2 Tbsp

shrimp, 1 lb (500 g) large, peeled and deveined

freshly ground pepper, ¼ tsp

olive oil, 1 Tbsp

canola oil, 1 Tbsp

feta cheese, ¼ cup (1½ oz/45 g) crumbled

MAKES 4 SERVINGS

1 In a large bowl, combine orange juice, 2 tablespoons of lime juice, and salt. Cut watermelon into quarters and remove rind. Cut fruit into cubes and add to juice mixture. Cut mint leaves lengthwise into thin ribbons. Add to bowl and stir gently to mix well. Cover and refrigerate until ready to serve.

2 Put shrimp in a bowl and sprinkle with pepper. Add olive oil and remaining 2 tablespoons lime juice and toss to coat. Refrigerate while you prepare grill.

3 Build a hot fire in a charcoal grill or preheat a gas grill to high. Brush grill rack with canola oil. Drain shrimp and thread onto 4 flat metal skewers. Grill shrimp directly over heat, turning once, until bright pink and opaque, 4–5 minutes total.

4 Remove watermelon mixture from refrigerator and gently stir in feta. Divide watermelon salad among 4 dinner plates. Push grilled shrimp off skewers onto each portion. Serve right away.

Low in fat and high in nutrients and flavor, watermelon deserves a place at the dinner table. If you're watching your sodium intake, omit the cheese.

watermelon
- Excellent source of vitamin C
- Contains lycopene, an antioxidant linked to cancer and heart disease prevention
- High water content helps keep you full

shrimp
- Excellent source of selenium, an antioxidant that boosts immunity
- Provides healthful omega-3 fatty acids

per serving 280 calories, 19 g protein, 30 g carbs, 10 g fat (2.5 g saturated fat), 150 mg cholesterol, 2 g fiber, 790 mg sodium

If you're lucky enough to have a source for freshly made corn tortillas, you'll want to use them in this recipe. If possible, purchase wild salmon rather than farmed—not only is it a more sustainable option, but it's more nutritious and flavorful, too.

SALMON TACOS WITH MANGO–AVOCADO SALSA

ripe avocado, 1

ripe mango, 1 large

red Fresno chile, 1, seeded and minced

red onion, 1/3 cup (2 oz/60 g) minced

fresh cilantro, 3 Tbsp chopped

fresh lime juice, 3 Tbsp

olive oil, 2 Tbsp

salt, 1/2 tsp

canola oil, 1 Tbsp

salmon fillet, 1 lb (500 g), skin and pin bones removed

freshly ground pepper, 1/4 tsp

soft corn tortillas, 8

radishes, 1/4 cup (1 oz/30 g) thinly sliced

MAKES 4 SERVINGS

Besides a little chopping, this superfood-packed recipe takes about 10 minutes to cook, making it an ideal dinner for any night of the week.

mangoes
- Outstanding source of blood pressure–lowering potassium
- Rich in vitamins A and C
- Known to aid digestion

avocados
- Excellent source of healthful monounsaturated fat
- Rich in cholesterol-lowering compounds
- Their healthy fat aids in the absorption of certain vitamins and plant compounds

per serving 470 calories, 27 g protein, 36 g carbs, 26 g fat (3.5 g saturated fat), 60 mg cholesterol, 7 g fiber, 370 mg sodium

1 Halve, pit, and peel avocado. Cut into small cubes and place in a large bowl.

2 Hold mango upright on a cutting board. Using a sharp chef's knife, make downward cuts along each flat side of pit to separate from flesh. Remove skin with a vegetable peeler and cut flesh into small cubes. Add to bowl with avocado, then add chile, onion, cilantro, lime juice, 1 tablespoon of olive oil, and 1/4 teaspoon of salt. Stir gently to mix well. Cover and refrigerate until ready to serve.

3 Build a medium-hot fire in a charcoal grill or preheat a gas grill to medium. Brush grill rack with canola oil. Place salmon on a plate and brush both sides lightly with remaining 1 tablespoon olive oil. Sprinkle both sides with remaining 1/4 teaspoon salt and pepper.

4 Grill salmon directly over heat until just cooked through, 3–5 minutes per side, depending on thickness of fillet. Transfer to a platter and cover loosely with aluminum foil. Wrap tortillas in another piece of foil and warm on grill until pliable, about 5 minutes.

5 To assemble, break the salmon into 8 pieces. Place 2 warm tortillas on each of 4 dinner plates and place a piece of salmon in center of each. Top each piece of salmon with salsa and radishes. Serve right away.

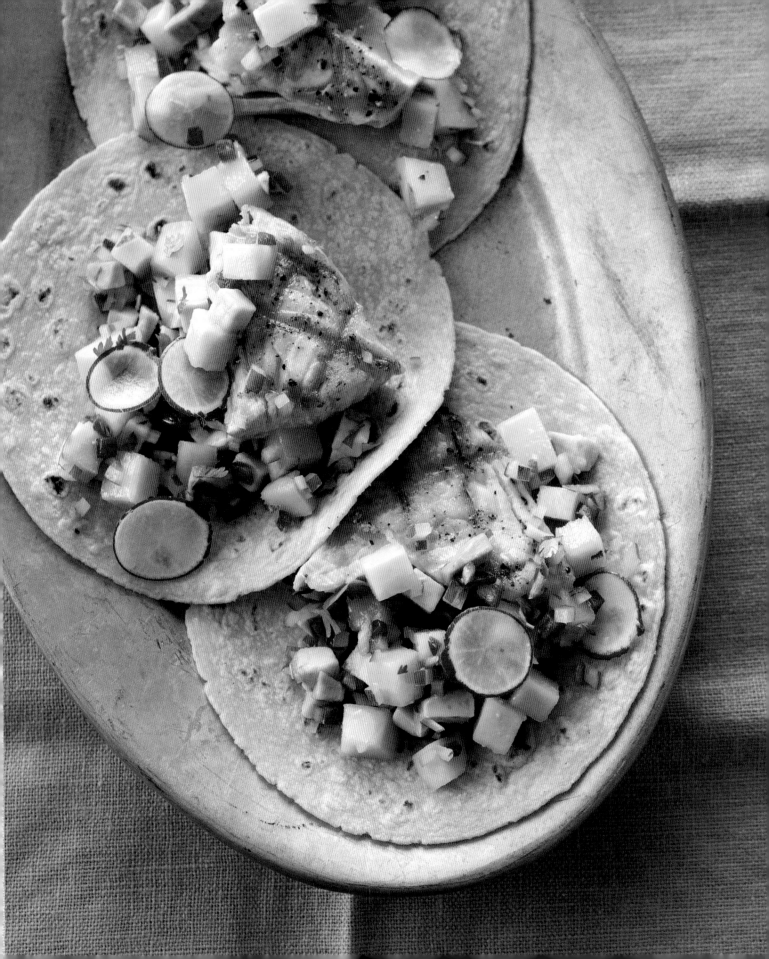

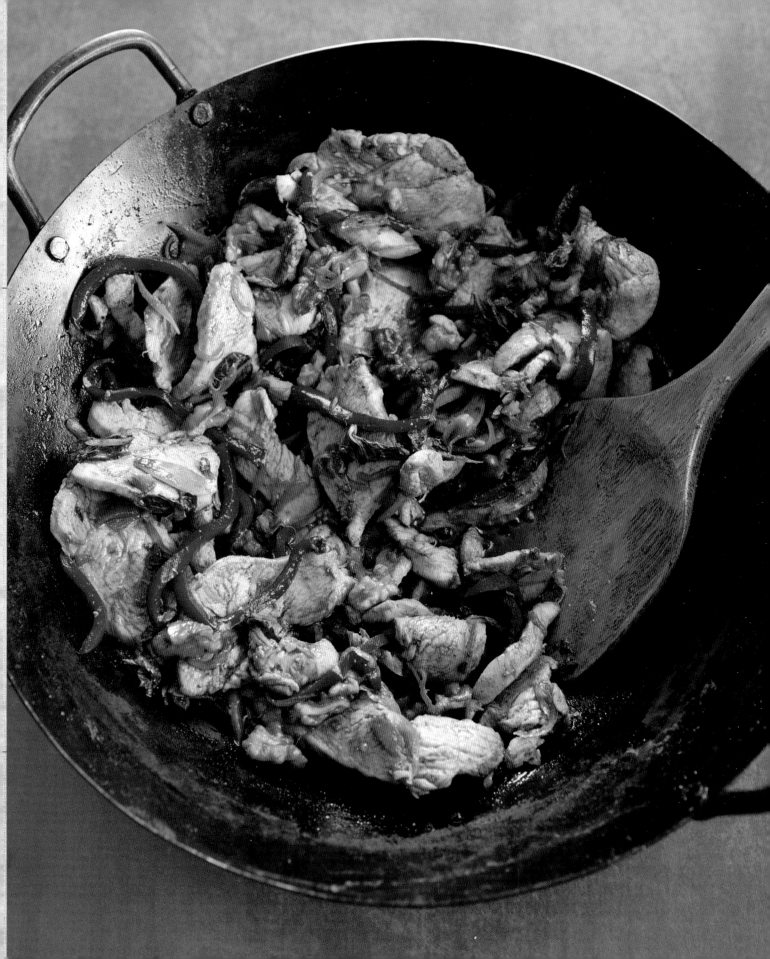

This super quick stir-fry is the perfect solution for a busy weeknight. If you don't own a wok, use a large, heavy frying pan, and make sure to heat the oil well before adding any ingredients. Use Thai basil, rather than Italian, if you can find it at the market.

WALNUT CHICKEN WITH BASIL

walnut pieces, ½ cup (2 oz/60 g)

low-sodium soy sauce, 3 Tbsp

fresh lime juice, 2 Tbsp

honey, 2 Tbsp

peanut oil, 3 tsp

red bell pepper, 1, seeded and thinly sliced

shallots, 2 large, thinly sliced

boneless, skinless chicken breast halves, 3 (about 5 oz/155 g each), thinly sliced across the grain

fresh basil leaves, ½ cup packed (½ oz/15 g) , torn into pieces

MAKES 4 SERVINGS

1 Preheat oven to 350°F (180°C). Spread walnuts on a baking sheet and toast until lightly browned and fragrant, about 10 minutes. Immediately pour onto a plate to cool. Set aside.

2 In a small bowl, whisk together soy sauce, lime juice, and honey. Set aside.

3 Heat 1½ teaspoons of oil in a wok over high heat. Add bell pepper and cook just until wilted, 1–2 minutes. Transfer bell pepper to a plate and add remaining 1½ teaspoons oil to pan. Add shallots and cook, stirring constantly, until just beginning to brown, 30 seconds–1 minute.

4 Add chicken to pan with shallots and cook, stirring often, until opaque throughout, 3–4 minutes. Return bell pepper to pan and stir in soy-sauce mixture, basil, and walnuts. Toss and stir just until basil is wilted, about 1 minute longer. Serve right away.

This one-pot dish boasts protein and nutrients without a lot of calories or carbs. Serve it over brown rice for a hearty, balanced meal.

chicken breast
- Quick-cooking lean protein
- Good source of B vitamins
- Choose skinless chicken breast to reduce saturated fat

walnuts
- Highest heart-healthy omega-3 fatty acids among nuts
- May help reduce cholesterol and improve brain health
- Source of disease-fighting antioxidants

per serving 310 calories, 26 g protein, 17 g carbs, 16 g fat (2 g saturated fat), 70 mg cholesterol, 2 g fiber, 530 mg sodium

You can adjust the amount of spice to suit your taste in this creamy, and always popular, Asian peanut sauce. Use a combination of colored bell peppers, such as red and yellow, for visual appeal. If you like, round out the meal with a side of tabbouleh (page 173).

GRILLED CHICKEN SKEWERS WITH SPICY PEANUT SAUCE

Bell peppers add color, flavor, and nutrients to these simple chicken skewers; a creamy peanut sauce provides a touch of richness.

peanut butter
- Its unique combination of protein, healthy fat, and fiber promotes fullness
- Rich in heart-smart monounsaturated fat
- Choose all-natural varieties without added sugar

bell peppers
- Excellent source of vitamin C
- Choose red, yellow, or orange peppers for the most antioxidant power

per serving 440 calories,
42 g protein, 14 g carbs,
24 g fat (4 g saturated fat),
110 mg cholesterol, 3 g fiber,
580 mg sodium

canola oil, 1 Tbsp
low-sodium creamy peanut butter, ⅓ cup (3½ oz/105 g)
light coconut milk, ⅓ cup (3 fl oz/90 ml)
fresh lime juice, 1½ Tbsp
light brown sugar, 1½ Tbsp firmly packed
low-sodium soy sauce, 3½ tsp
Asian red chile paste, 1½ tsp

boneless, skinless chicken breasts, 1½ lb (750 g), cut into 1½-inch (4-cm) chunks
bell peppers, 2, seeded and cut into 1½-inch (4-cm) chunks
olive oil, 1 Tbsp
sea salt, ¼ tsp
freshly ground pepper, ¼ tsp

MAKES 4 SERVINGS

1 Build a hot fire in a charcoal grill or preheat a gas grill to medium-high. Brush grill rack with canola oil.

2 In a bowl, whisk together peanut butter, coconut milk, lime juice, brown sugar, soy sauce, and red chile paste. Transfer sauce to a serving bowl or bowls and set aside.

3 Thread chicken and bell pepper pieces alternately onto 8 metal or soaked wooden skewers, dividing them evenly. Lightly brush with olive oil and sprinkle with salt and pepper.

4 Grill skewers directly over heat until chicken is nicely grill-marked on first side, about 3 minutes. Turn and grill until chicken is browned on second side and opaque throughout, 2–3 minutes longer. Remove from grill and serve right away, with peanut sauce for dipping.

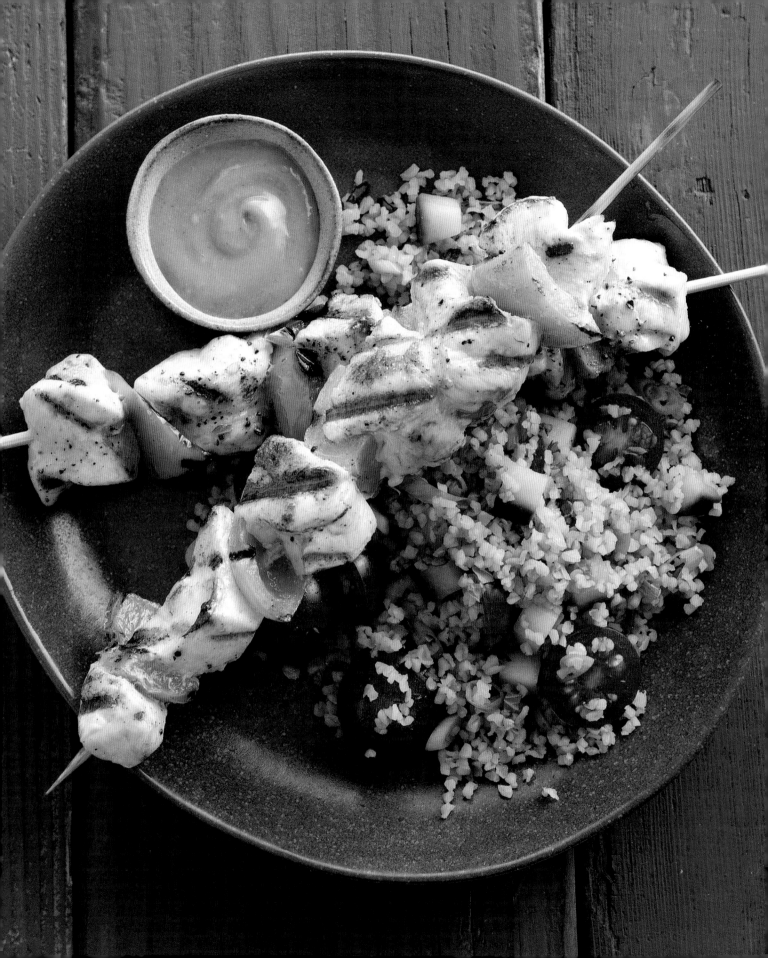

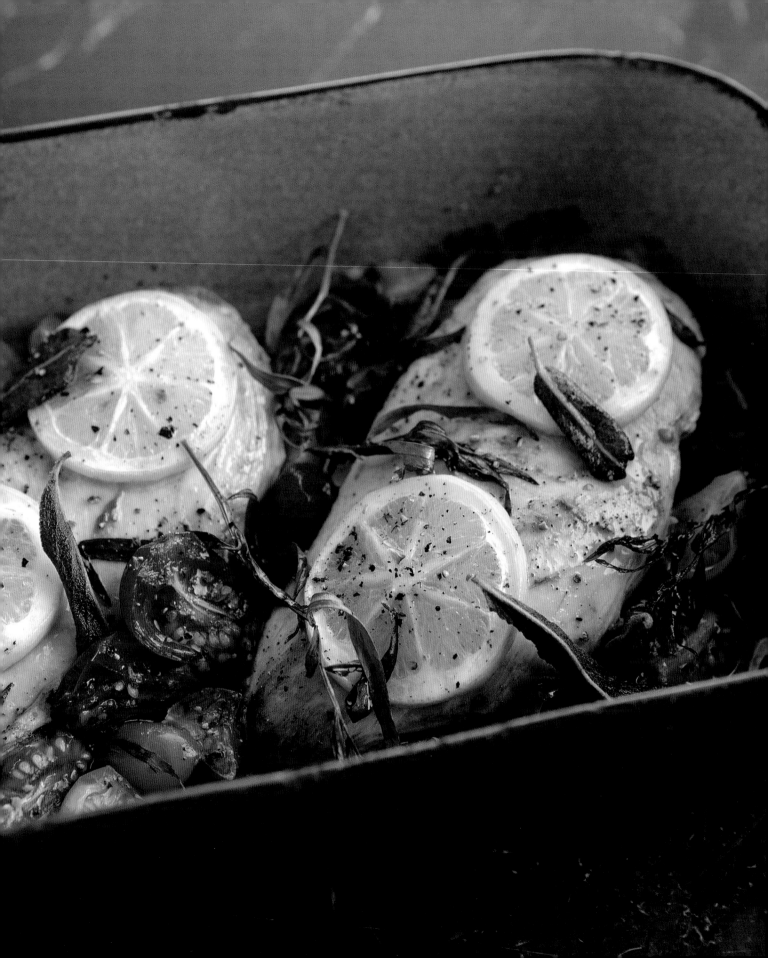

Cherry tomatoes become even sweeter as they bake, making them a tasty accompaniment to chicken breasts that cook right alongside. If desired, you can omit the tarragon and sage and top the finished dish with fresh basil and parsley leaves lightly drizzled with olive oil.

BAKED CHICKEN WITH CHERRY TOMATOES, HERBS & LEMON

olive oil, 6½ tsp

boneless, skinless chicken breast halves, 4 (about 5 oz/155 g each)

cherry or grape tomatoes, 8 oz (250 g), halved

balsamic vinegar, 1½ tsp

sea salt, ½ tsp

freshly ground pepper, to taste

lemon, 1, cut into 8 thin slices

fresh tarragon sprigs, 6–8

fresh sage leaves, 8–10

MAKES 4 SERVINGS

1 Preheat oven to 375°F (190°C). Lightly grease a baking dish with 2 teaspoons of olive oil.

2 Place chicken in prepared baking dish. Arrange tomatoes around chicken. Drizzle chicken and tomatoes with vinegar and 2½ teaspoons of olive oil. Sprinkle with salt and pepper.

3 Top each chicken breast half with 2 lemon slices. Arrange tarragon sprigs and sage leaves over and around chicken. Drizzle remaining 2 teaspoons olive oil over herbs.

4 Bake until chicken is opaque throughout, 25–30 minutes. Arrange a chicken breast on each of 4 plates, spooning equal amounts of tomatoes and herbs around each. Drizzle with some pan juices and serve right away.

Here's a low-fat, low-fuss way to enjoy tender chicken breast. Baking the chicken takes longer than sautéing or poaching, but it produces more flavorful meat.

cherry tomatoes
- Excellent source of vitamins A and C
- High in lycopene, which is thought to protect against cancer and heart disease
- Store at room temperature for best flavor

lemons
- Excellent source of vitamin C
- Contain compounds that have antioxidant and anti-cancer properties

per serving 240 calories, 31 g protein, 5 g carbs, 11 g fat (2 g saturated fat), 90 mg cholesterol, 2 g fiber, 410 mg sodium

Chipotles are smoked, pickled jalapeño chiles. To make chipotle purée, in a blender or food processor, whirl the contents of a 7-oz (220-g) can of chipotle chiles in adobo sauce until smooth. Transfer to an airtight container and store in the refrigerator for up to 3 weeks.

GRILLED STEAK, BELL PEPPER & ONION FAJITAS

To curb the overall fat, reduce the amount of steak to 12 oz (375 g) and omit the avocado.

flank steak
- Excellent source of iron, zinc, and selenium
- Rich in protein

napa cabbage
- Excellent source of folate for heart health
- Strongly linked to cancer prevention
- Serve fresh to retain cancer-preventing nutrients

per serving 510 calories, 43 g protein, 57 g carbs, 20 g fat (4.5 g saturated fat), 70 mg cholesterol, 9 g fiber, 800 mg sodium

flank steak, 1 lb (500 g)

fresh lime juice, ¼ cup (2 fl oz/60 ml) plus 2 Tbsp

fresh orange juice, ¼ cup (2 fl oz/60 ml)

garlic cloves, 2, smashed

olive oil, 2 Tbsp

chipotle chile purée, 1½ tsp (see note)

sea salt, ½ tsp plus a pinch

napa cabbage, ¼ head, cored and thinly sliced (about 2 cups/6 oz/185 g)

radishes, 3, thinly sliced

fresh cilantro, 1 Tbsp chopped

red, orange, or yellow bell peppers, or a combination, 3, seeded and sliced lengthwise into thick strips

red onion, 1, cut into slices ¾ inch (2 cm) thick

whole-wheat tortillas, 8 (6 inches/15 cm in diameter)

ripe avocado, 1, pitted, peeled, and diced

MAKES 8 FAJITAS; 4 SERVINGS

1. Trim fat from steak. In a bowl, whisk together ¼ cup lime juice, orange juice, garlic, 1 tablespoon of olive oil, chipotle purée, and ½ teaspoon salt. Place steak in bowl with marinade and turn to coat. Cover and let marinate in refrigerator for at least 15 minutes and up to 4 hours.

2. Build a hot fire in a charcoal grill or preheat a gas grill to medium-high.

3. In a large bowl, toss cabbage, radishes, and cilantro with 2 tablespoons lime juice. Set aside.

4. Put peppers and onion in a bowl and sprinkle with remaining 1 tablespoon olive oil and a pinch of salt. Grill, turning as needed, until vegetables are tender and nicely browned, 6–8 minutes total. Transfer to a large platter.

5. Remove steak from bowl and discard marinade. Arrange steak on grill directly over heat and cook, turning once, for 4–6 minutes total for medium-rare. Transfer to a platter and let rest for 10 minutes. Wrap tortillas in a piece of foil and place on grill over indirect heat to warm.

6. Carve steak across grain into thin slices. Serve with grilled vegetables, warm tortillas, cabbage mixture, and avocado, letting diners assemble their fajitas.

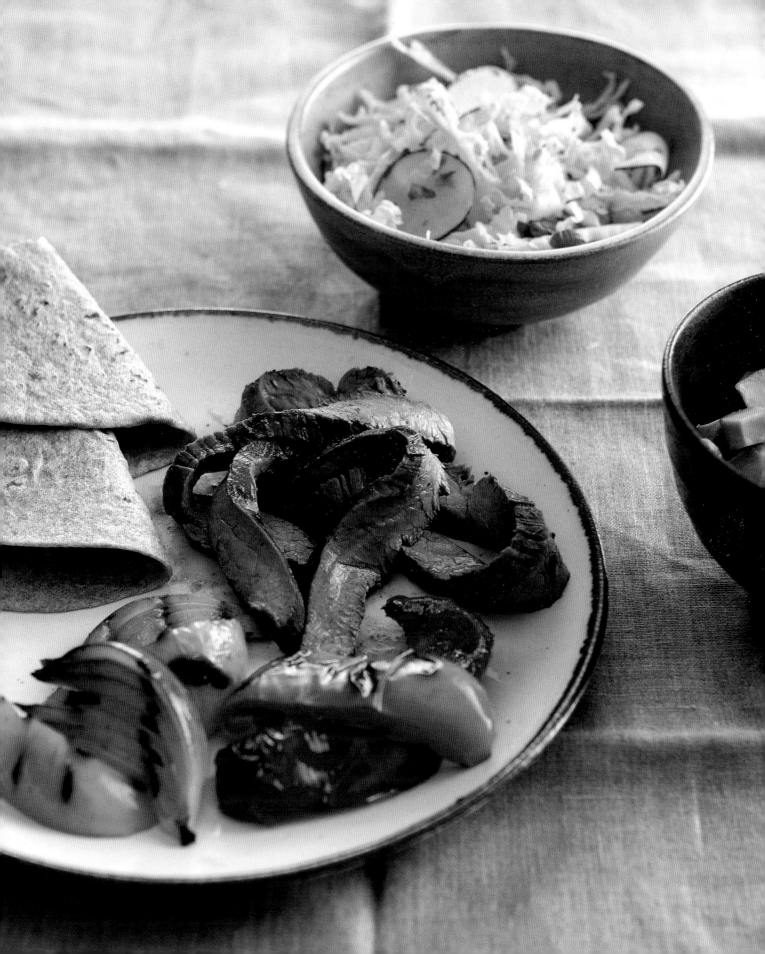

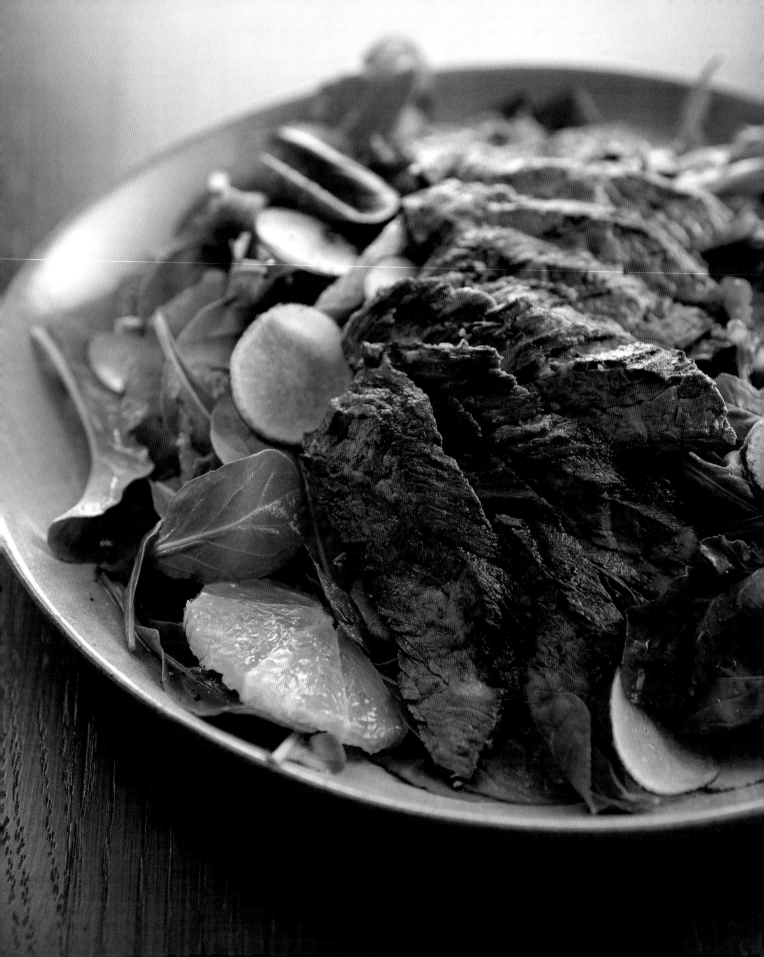

This flavor-packed salad is quick enough for a casual weeknight meal, but elegant enough for your next dinner party. For a tropical twist, substitute pineapple for the oranges. Skirt steak is relatively lean, and cooks quickly; if you prefer, you can grill it (see page 142).

STEAK & ARUGULA SALAD WITH ORANGES

skirt steak, 1 lb (500 g)
low-sodium soy sauce, ¼ cup (2 fl oz/60 ml)
fresh orange juice, 4 Tbsp (2 fl oz/60 ml)
fresh lime juice, 4 Tbsp (2 fl oz/60 ml)
fresh ginger, 1 Tbsp minced
garlic, 1 clove, pressed or minced

oranges, 2
extra-virgin olive oil, 2 Tbsp
baby arugula, 4 cups (4 oz/125 g)
radishes, 4, trimmed and sliced
freshly ground pepper, to taste

MAKES 4 SERVINGS

1 Trim fat from steak and cut into 2 or 3 pieces.

2 In a zippered plastic bag, combine soy sauce, orange juice, 1 tablespoon of lime juice, ginger, and garlic. Add steak, seal tightly, and turn to mix marinade and coat steak. Refrigerate for at least 1 hour and up to overnight.

3 Preheat broiler. Remove steak from bag and discard marinade. Place steak on a broiler pan and place about 2 inches (5 cm) from heat source. Broil, turning once, for about 8 minutes total for medium-rare.

4 Meanwhile, using a sharp knife, cut a thin slice off both ends of each orange, then cut away peel and bitter white pith, following fruit's curve. Cut orange in half lengthwise, then slice crosswise into thin half-moons.

5 In a large bowl, mix remaining 3 tablespoons lime juice and olive oil. Add arugula, oranges, and radishes and toss to mix well. Mound on a platter. Carve steak across grain into slices ¼ inch (6 mm) thick and arrange over salad. Sprinkle with pepper and serve right away.

To lower the fat in the salad, reduce the steak to 12 oz (375 g). Or, slice or cube 8 oz (250 g) firm tofu, and marinate and cook it as you would the steak.

oranges
- Excellent source of vitamin C
- Contain nutrients linked to heart health, such as folate and potassium
- Rich in cancer-preventing compounds

garlic
- A natural blood thinner
- May protect against some forms of cancer

per serving 340 calories, 24 g protein, 11 g carbs, 22 g fat (7 g saturated fat), 70 mg cholesterol, 2 g fiber, 210 mg sodium

This hearty stir-fry is the ultimate one-dish meal. Swap in other quick-cooking vegetables, like broccoli florets, snow peas, or asparagus, if you like. Pork tenderloin is easier to slice for stir-frying if you chill it first in the freezer for about 30 minutes.

STIR-FRIED PORK & BOK CHOY

This dish is deliciously simple, highlighting a lean, quick-cooking protein, a nutrient-rich vegetable, and a few Asian-inspired flavorings like ginger, garlic, and soy sauce.

bok choy
- High in folate and vitamins A and C
- Packed with nutrients thought to detoxify and fight cancer

red pepper flakes
- High in capsaicin, known for its anti-inflammatory and pain-relief properties
- May boost metabolism and reduce risk of type 2 diabetes

per serving 290 calories, 26 g protein, 28 g carbs, 7 g fat (1.5 g saturated fat), 75 mg cholesterol, 4 g fiber, 290 mg sodium

dry sherry, 2 Tbsp
low-sodium soy sauce, 1 Tbsp
Asian red chile paste, ½ tsp
baby bok choy, 1 lb (500 g)
pork tenderloin, 1 lb (500 g)
peanut oil, 3 tsp

garlic, 2 cloves, pressed or minced
fresh ginger, 1 Tbsp minced or grated
red pepper flakes, ¼ tsp
cooked brown rice, 2 cups (10 oz/315 g)

MAKES 4 SERVINGS

1 In a small bowl, stir together sherry, soy sauce, and chile paste and set aside.

2 Trim stem ends from baby bok choy and separate into leaves. Cut pork tenderloin crosswise into ½-inch (12-mm) slices, and then cut into 1-inch (2.5-cm) strips.

3 Heat 1½ teaspoons of oil in a wok or large nonstick frying pan over high heat. When oil is hot, add bok choy and toss and stir just until crisp-tender, about 2 minutes. Transfer to a bowl.

4 Add remaining 1½ teaspoons oil to pan. When hot, add garlic and ginger and cook, stirring constantly, until fragrant but not browned, 15–30 seconds. Add pork to pan and cook, stirring, until lightly browned and cooked through, 2–3 minutes longer.

5 Return bok choy to pan along with any juices accumulated in bowl, then add sherry mixture and toss and stir just until heated through, about 1 minute. Sprinkle with chile flakes and serve right away with rice.

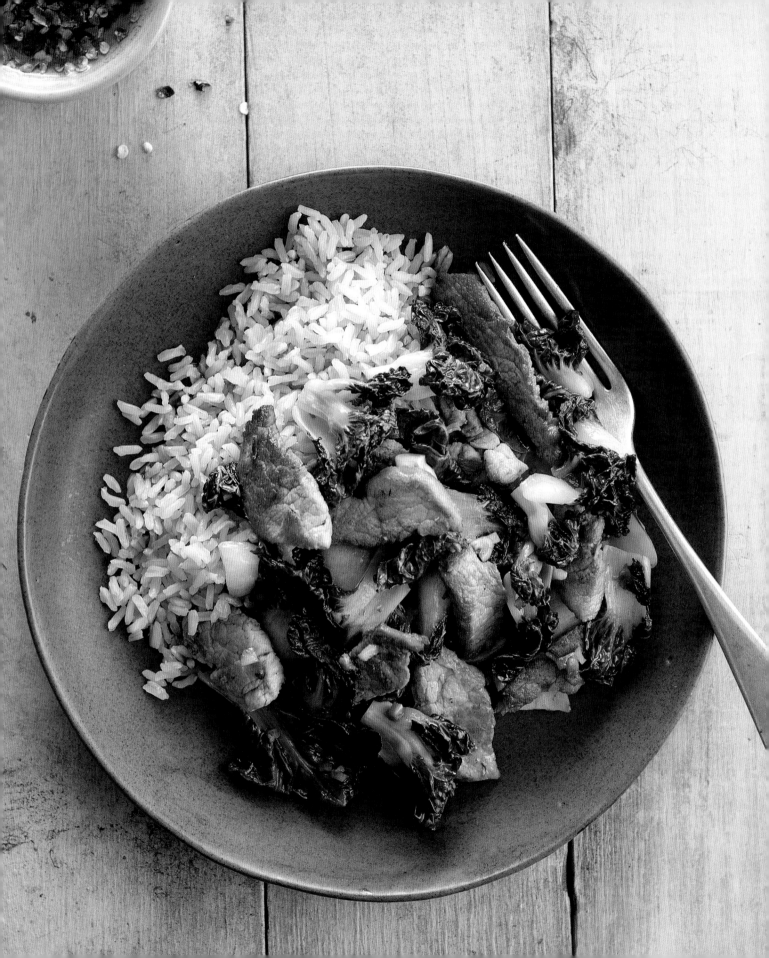

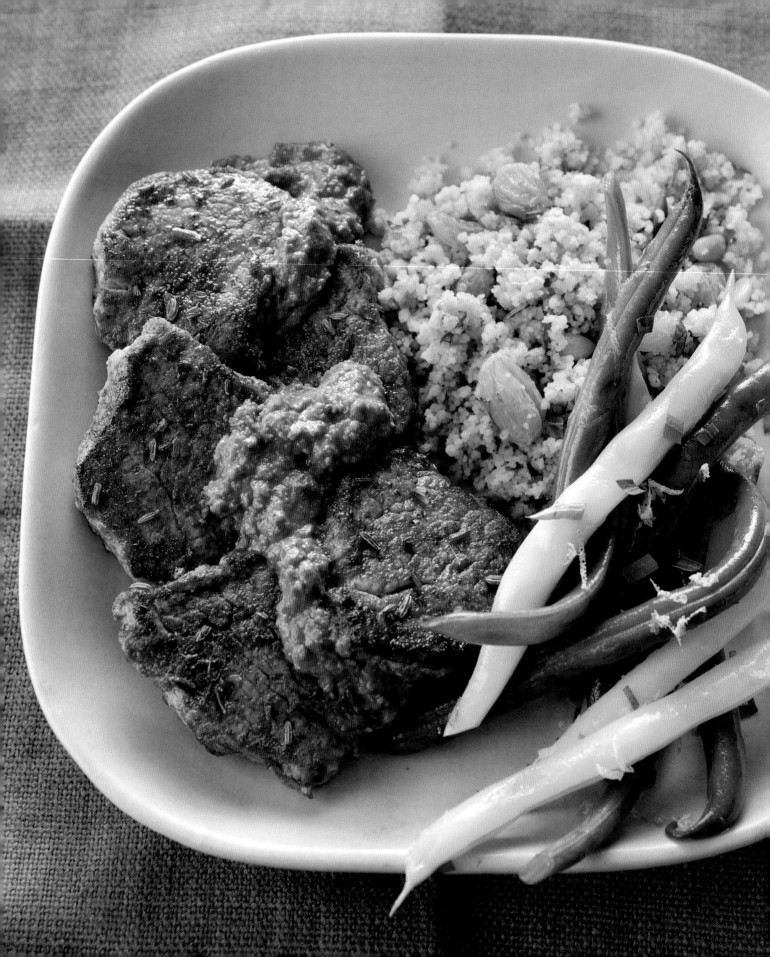

Pork tenderloin is both tender and lean, so take care not to overcook it—the center of the pork should be just barely rosy when it is done. To round out the meal, serve with sautéed seasonal vegetables and a simple grain side dish, like couscous.

PORK MEDALLIONS WITH ROMESCO SAUCE

pork tenderloin, 1 lb (500 g)

walnut pieces, ¼ cup (1 oz/30 g)

crushed fennel seed, ½ tsp

ground cumin, ½ tsp

salt, ¾ tsp

smoked paprika, 2 tsp

garlic, 1 clove, chopped

roasted red bell peppers, jarred or homemade (page 214), 1½ cups (8½ oz/265 g) drained, liquid reserved

extra-virgin olive oil, 4 Tbsp (2 fl oz/60 ml)

dry sherry or red wine vinegar, 1 Tbsp

cayenne pepper, ¼ tsp

MAKES 4 SERVINGS

1 Preheat oven to 350°F (180°C). Trim fat and any silvery membrane from tenderloin and cut crosswise into rounds about ½ inch (12 mm) thick.

2 Spread walnuts on a baking sheet and toast until lightly browned and fragrant, about 10 minutes. Immediately pour onto a plate to cool.

3 In a small bowl, stir together fennel seed, cumin, ½ teaspoon of salt, and ½ teaspoon of paprika. Rub spice mixture into both sides of pork rounds and let stand at room temperature while you make the sauce.

4 In a blender or food processor, combine walnuts and garlic and process until finely chopped. Add roasted peppers, 2 tablespoons of olive oil, sherry, remaining 1½ teaspoons paprika, cayenne, and remaining ¼ teaspoon salt and whirl until smooth. Stir in up to 1 tablespoon roasted-pepper liquid if sauce is too thick. Set aside.

5 Heat remaining 2 tablespoons olive oil in a large frying pan over medium heat. Working in batches if necessary, add pork loin rounds to pan in a single layer and cook just until browned and still faintly pink in the center, about 2 minutes per side. Transfer to a platter and let rest for about 5 minutes.

6 Divide pork among 4 dinner plates and spoon *romesco* sauce over meat. Serve right away.

For a lower-fat dish that's still big on flavor, serve the pork with applesauce (page 215) instead of the *romesco*.

pork tenderloin
- Quick-cooking complete protein that's as lean as skinless chicken breast
- Outstanding source of thiamin, needed to convert carbohydrates to energy

extra-virgin olive oil
- Linked to prevention of cancer, dementia, and heart disease
- One of nature's richest sources of monounsaturated fats
- Contains compounds that maintain blood vessel health

per serving 380 calories, 26 g protein, 6 g carbs, 29 g fat (4 g saturated fat), 75 mg cholesterol, 2 g fiber, 520 mg sodium

Premade whole-wheat pizza dough, available in the refrigerated section of many supermarkets, makes it easy to throw together a pizza that's healthy and infinitely better than takeout. Experiment with other fresh seasonal vegetable and herb toppings.

WHOLE-WHEAT PIZZA WITH BROCCOLI RABE & TURKEY SAUSAGE

If you're going to indulge in pizza, make your own using whole-wheat flour and nutritious toppings.

broccoli rabe
- Rich in cancer-preventing compounds
- Excellent source of vitamin K for bone health
- Steaming or blanching can help decrease bitter flavor

part-skim mozzarella
- Good source of calcium for strong bones and blood-pressure reduction
- Rich in protein
- Lower in fat and calories than most cheeses

per serving 480 calories, 23 g protein, 50 g carbs, 24 g fat (4.5 g saturated fat), 100 mg cholesterol, 11 g fiber, 1000 mg sodium

olive oil, 2 tsp plus 2 Tbsp
cornmeal, for dusting
whole-wheat pizza dough, 1 lb (500 g)
turkey sausages, 2
garlic, 1 clove, pressed or minced
red pepper flakes, ¼ tsp

broccoli rabe, 1 bunch, trimmed and coarsely chopped
sea salt, ⅛ tsp
part-skim mozzarella cheese, ½ cup (2 oz/60 g) shredded

MAKES ONE 12-INCH (30-CM) PIZZA; 4 SERVINGS

1 Place a rack in lowest position in oven and preheat to 400°F (200°C). Grease a baking sheet or 12-inch (30-cm) pizza pan with 2 teaspoons of olive oil and dust with cornmeal.

2 On a lightly floured work surface, pat and stretch dough into a 12-inch (30-cm) round. Transfer to prepared baking sheet and set aside.

3 Heat 1 tablespoon of olive oil in a frying pan over medium heat. Turn sausage out of its casings into pan and cook, stirring constantly and using spoon to break up meat, until lightly browned on all sides, 3–5 minutes. Transfer to a plate and scrape out any browned bits from pan.

4 Add remaining 1 tablespoon olive oil to pan. Add garlic and red pepper flakes and cook just until fragrant, about 1 minute. Add broccoli rabe (carefully, as any water clinging to broccoli rabe may cause oil to splatter) and sprinkle with salt. Cook, stirring often, until bright green and evenly coated with oil, about 2 minutes. Add 2 tablespoons water to pan and steam until tender, about 5 minutes longer. (Sprinkle up to 2 tablespoons more water if needed.)

5 Scatter cheese, broccoli rabe, and sausage evenly on top of dough. Bake until crust is golden brown on edges and cheese is bubbling, 15–18 minutes. Let cool slightly, then cut into squares or wedges and serve right away.

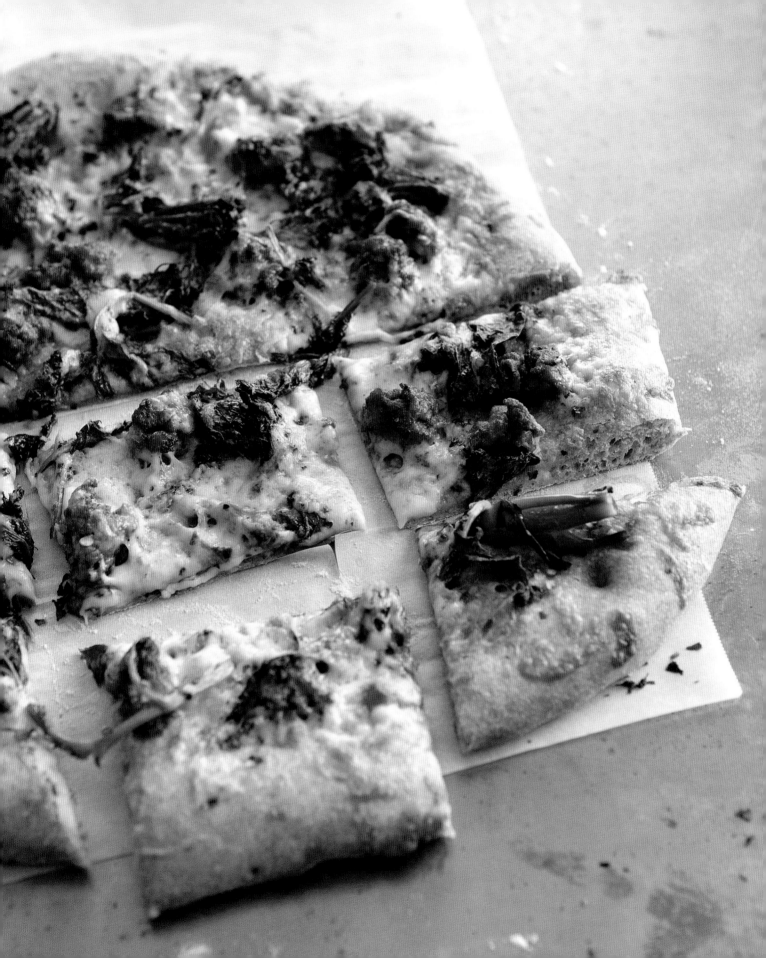

Nutritious side dishes are the ideal opportunity to round out your diet and sneak in foods that you may not otherwise get enough of, like fruits, vegetables, and whole grains.

SIDES

QUICK-FIX IDEAS FOR SIDES

COOK IT IN A FLASH

GARLIC SPINACH Cut a bunch of spinach, including the tender stems, crosswise into wide strips and sauté in olive oil over medium heat just until wilted, about 30 seconds. Add 2 cloves garlic, minced, and a splash of water. Cook, stirring, until tender, just a few seconds longer. Season to taste with salt and pepper and serve with lemon wedges for squeezing.

ROASTED MUSHROOMS Arrange white or cremini mushrooms, stem side up, in a lightly greased baking dish. Drizzle with a little olive oil and sprinkle with fresh thyme or sage leaves. Roast at 375°F (190°C), stirring occasionally, until the mushrooms are juicy and tender, 10–15 minutes. Season lightly with salt and pepper.

SWEET POTATO MASH Peel and quarter sweet potatoes and place in a saucepan with water to cover. Bring the water to a boil over high heat, then reduce the heat to medium-low, cover, and simmer until the potatoes are tender, 15–20 minutes. Drain, transfer to a bowl, and mash. Season with salt, pepper, and a splash of orange juice.

NO COOKING NEEDED

CRUNCHY SLAWS Shred or thinly slice a combination of colorful, crunchy vegetables and toss with a simple dressing for the perfect barbecue or picnic side. Try one of these combinations (or create your own): cabbage, carrot, fresh dill or dill seeds, and buttermilk dressing; apple, fennel, radicchio, walnuts, and lemon-honey dressing; napa cabbage, jicama, fresh cilantro, and ginger-lime dressing.

TOSSED GREEN SALAD Use this basic vinaigrette to dress any greens you have available: In a jar with a tight-fitting lid, combine 2 tablespoons red or white wine vinegar, 2 teaspoons Dijon mustard, and ½ teaspoon salt. Add ¼ cup (2 fl oz/60 ml) extra-virgin olive oil, cover, and shake to combine. Season with freshly ground pepper. Adjust the flavorings by using balsamic vinegar or fresh lemon juice in place of the red or white wine vinegar, or adding minced garlic, herbs, or anchovies to taste.

MAKE IT AHEAD

COOKED DRIED BEANS Soak dried beans before cooking them for the best flavor and texture (see page 214). Drain the beans and place in a saucepan with water to cover by about 4 inches (10 cm). Bring to a boil over high heat, then reduce the heat to low, cover partially, and simmer until tender but not mushy, 1–3 hours, depending on the variety and age of the beans. Season with salt. Let cool completely in their cooking liquid, then drain and store in an airtight container or zippered plastic bag in the refrigerator for up to 3 days or in the freezer for up to 3 months. Reheat and serve as a simple side, or add to soups, salads, or burritos.

COOKED BROWN RICE Combine 2 parts water with 1 part brown rice and a pinch of salt in a saucepan over high heat, and bring to a boil. Reduce the heat to low, cover, and simmer gently until the water is absorbed, 40–45 minutes. Spread the rice out on a baking sheet and let cool completely, then store in an airtight container or zippered plastic bag in the refrigerator for up to 3 days or in the freezer for up to 3 months. Reheat and serve with seafood, stir-fries, or curries.

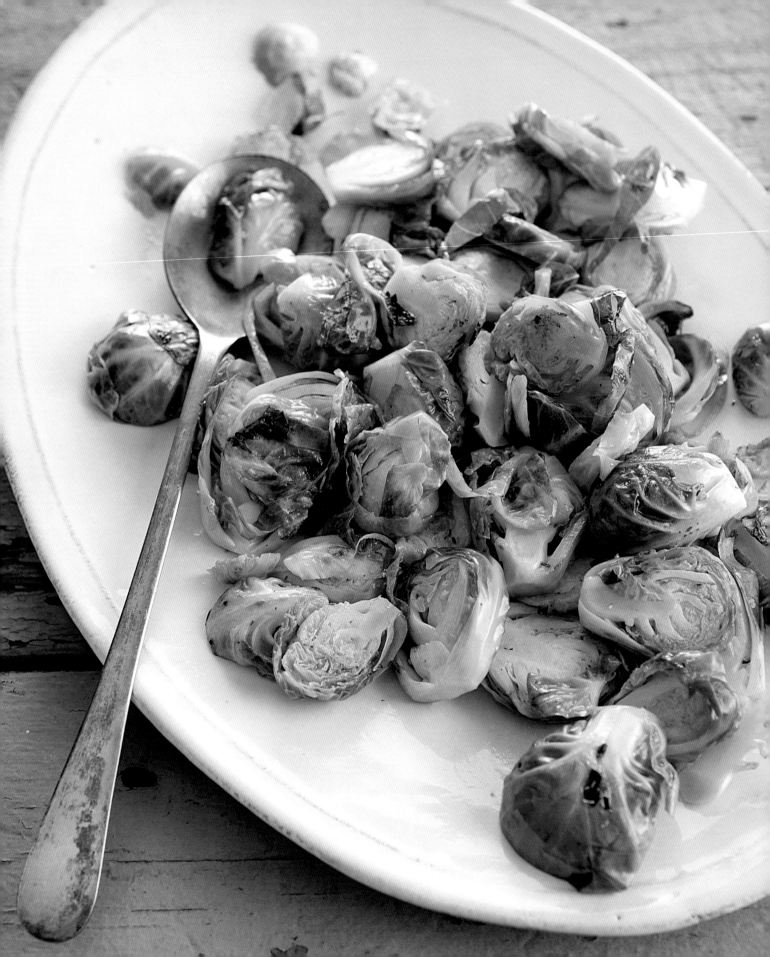

One way to bring out the best in Brussels sprouts is to cook them simply, with nothing more than a little good olive oil, lemon, and sea salt. Use the largest frying pan you have so the Brussels sprouts have room, to encourage even browning and crisp edges.

SAUTÉED BRUSSELS SPROUTS WITH LEMON

Brussels sprouts, 1 lb (500 g)

olive oil, 2 Tbsp

lemon zest strips, from ½ lemon, plus 3 Tbsp fresh lemon juice

sea salt, ¼ tsp

freshly ground pepper

MAKES 4 SERVINGS

1 Trim stem ends off Brussels sprouts and cut lengthwise into thin slices about ¼ inch (6 mm) thick.

2 Heat olive oil in a large frying pan over medium-high heat. When oil is hot, add sprouts, lemon zest, salt, and a few grindings of pepper. Cook, stirring often and keeping heat high but adjusting as needed to prevent scorching, until leaves are lightly browned around edges and tender, 7–8 minutes.

3 Stir in lemon juice and cook for 1 minute longer. Serve right away.

Sure, you can steam Brussels sprouts without adding any fat, but sautéing them in just a little bit of oil allows the vegetables to caramelize, which brings out their natural sugars and gives them appealing browned edges.

brussels sprouts
- Loaded with folate and vitamins C and K
- Filled with compounds that are thought to detoxify and protect against cancer
- Rich in fiber

per serving 110 calories, 4 g protein, 11 g carbs, 7 g fat (1 g saturated fat), 0 mg cholesterol, 4 g fiber, 150 mg sodium

This is a supremely simple preparation for kabocha, the dense, sweet winter squash sometimes referred to as Japanese pumpkin. Use a top-quality balsamic for the right balance of sweetness. Lining your baking pan with aluminum foil will ease cleanup.

BALSAMIC–ROASTED KABOCHA SQUASH

kabocha squash, 1, about 2½ lb
(1.25 kg)

olive oil, 2 Tbsp

sea salt, ¼ tsp

freshly ground pepper

balsamic vinegar, 2 Tbsp

MAKES 4 SERVINGS

There's no need to slather squash with butter, sugar, or maple syrup. Roasting will bring out the sweetness, and balsamic vinegar adds a perfectly suited tangy element.

kabocha squash

- Rich in beta-carotene, an antioxidant that the body converts to vitamin A
- Contains compounds that fight inflammation
- Excellent source of vitamins A and C

per serving 160 calories,
2 g protein, 24 g carbs,
8 g fat (1 g saturated fat),
0 mg cholesterol, 7 g fiber,
150 mg sodium

1 Preheat oven to 400°F (200°C).

2 Using a large chef's knife, cut squash in half lengthwise. Scoop out seeds and slice flesh crosswise into wedges ½–¾ inch (12 mm–2 cm) thick. Trim peel from each wedge.

3 Put squash on a baking pan, drizzle with olive oil, and toss to coat. Arrange in a single layer. Sprinkle with salt and a few grindings of pepper. Roast until tender when pierced, stirring twice to brown squash evenly, 15–18 minutes.

4 Drizzle squash with vinegar, return to oven, and continue roasting until vinegar has evaporated, about 3 minutes longer. Let cool slightly, then serve right away.

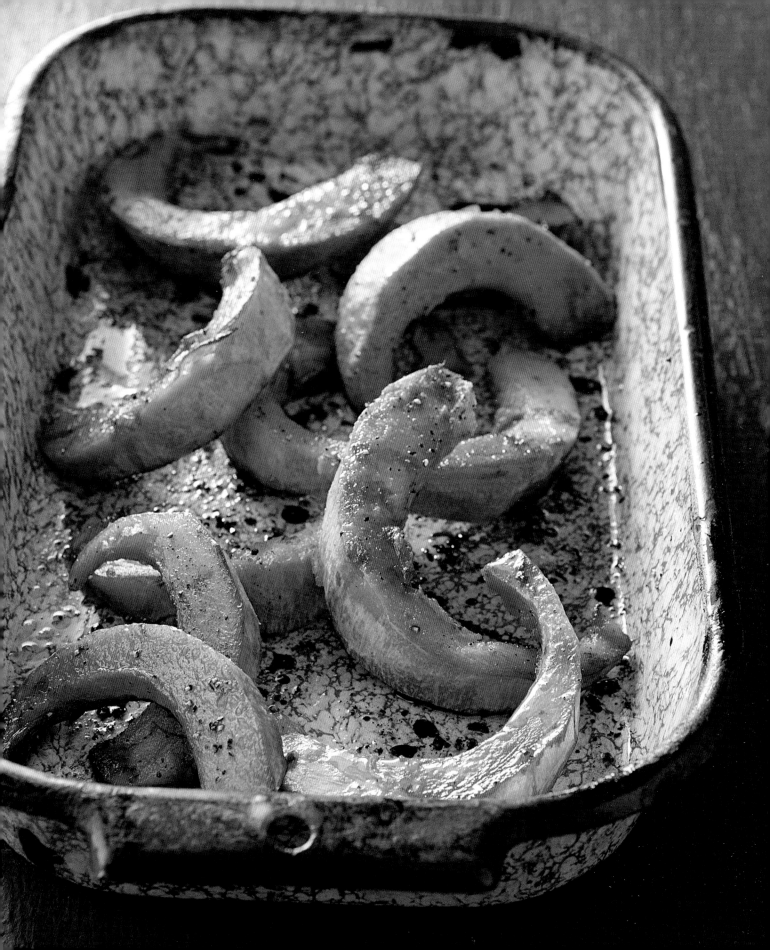

This side dish may be a revelation to you if you don't care for boiled or steamed broccoli; roasting brings out a deliciously sweet flavor, and the mustard–balsamic dressing adds pleasant tang. Buy pretrimmed broccoli florets to save time; you'll need about 1½ lb (750 g).

ROASTED BROCCOLI WITH PINE NUTS

A nutritional powerhouse, broccoli is recommended by nutritionists worldwide as one of the most healthful vegetables. It cooks fast, too, making it a great, go-to side dish.

broccoli

- Provides nutrients linked to bone health, such as calcium, vitamin K, and potassium
- Contains cancer-preventing compounds
- Excellent source of vitamin C

per serving
150 calories, 5 g protein, 12 g carbs, 11 g fat (1.5 g saturated fat), 0 mg cholesterol, 4 g fiber, 160 mg sodium

broccoli, 1–2 heads (about 2 lb/1 kg total weight)
pine nuts, ¼ cup (1 oz/30 g)
olive oil, 3 Tbsp
salt, ¼ tsp
balsamic vinegar, 2 Tbsp
Dijon mustard, 1 tsp

MAKES 6 SERVINGS

1 Preheat oven to 400°F (200°C). Cut broccoli into 1-inch (2.5-cm) florets.

2 In a small, dry frying pan over medium heat, toast pine nuts, stirring constantly, until lightly browned and fragrant, about 5 minutes. Immediately pour onto a plate to cool. Set aside.

3 In a large roasting pan, toss broccoli with 2 tablespoons of olive oil and salt until well coated. Spread in pan in a single layer. Roast, stirring two or three times, until browned and tender, 18–25 minutes.

4 In a large bowl, stir together vinegar, mustard, and remaining 1 tablespoon olive oil. Add warm broccoli and pine nuts and stir to coat well. Taste and adjust seasoning. Serve right away.

Asian greens are flavorful, with a pleasingly bitter edge. Use any combination of Chinese mustard greens, bok choy, or choy sum in this simple preparation. Serve them with poached salmon (page 214), seared scallops (page 128), or marinated skirt steak (page 145).

PAN-STEAMED ASIAN GREENS

Asian greens, 1 lb (500 g), trimmed

olive oil, 2 tsp

toasted sesame oil, 1 tsp

garlic, 1 clove, pressed or minced

low-sodium soy sauce, 1 tsp

MAKES 4 SERVINGS

1 Trim ends or any tough spines off greens and cut leaves crosswise into strips about 1½ inches (4 cm) wide. Transfer to a colander and rinse under cold running water. Drain well.

2 Heat both oils in a large frying pan over medium heat. Add garlic and stir until fragrant but not browned, about 30 seconds. Add greens and ¼ cup (2 fl oz/60 ml) water. Cover and cook, shaking pan occasionally, until greens are tender, 3–4 minutes. Remove from heat and stir in soy sauce. Serve right away.

Mellow the assertive flavor of hearty Asian cooking greens, such as mustard greens, with a dressing of healthy oils and aromatic garlic. A splash of low-sodium soy sauce adds just the right touch of saltiness.

mustard greens

- A member of the cruciferous vegetable family
- Excellent source of folate and vitamins A, C, and K
- Contain compounds that promote heart health

per serving 60 calories, 2 g protein, 5 g carbs, 3.5 g fat (0 g saturated fat), 0 mg cholesterol, 3 g fiber, 105 mg sodium

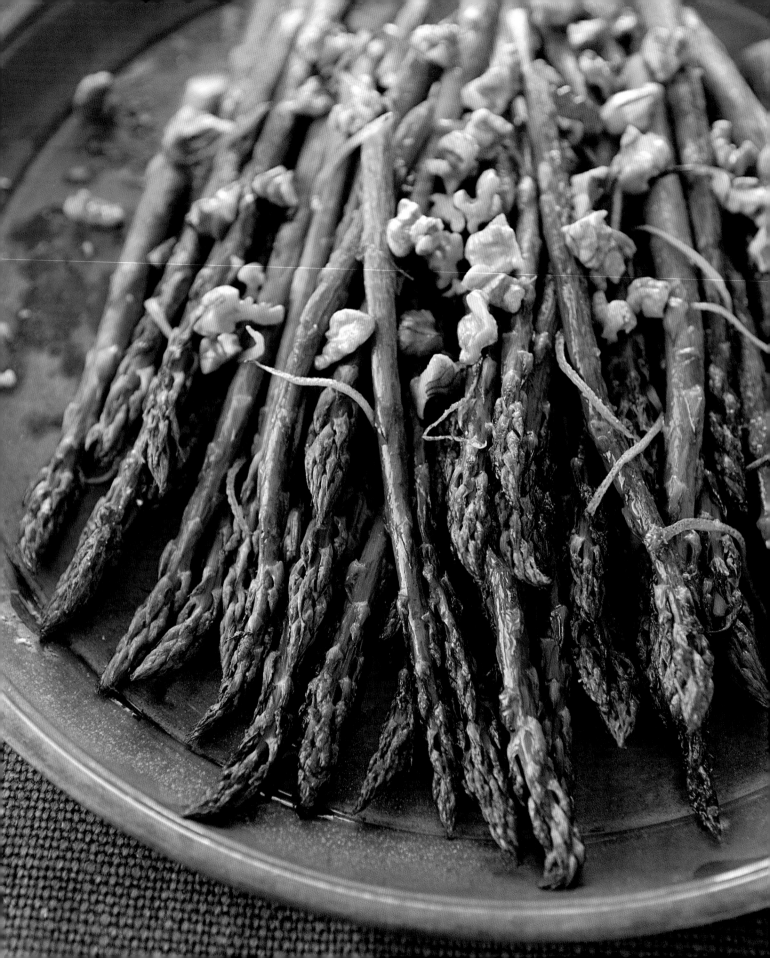

This quick spring side dish brings together three elements that make a beautiful composition on the plate. Pair it with chicken or fish. The orange zest will caramelize deliciously—stir it once or twice during the roasting time to keep it from burning.

ROASTED ASPARAGUS WITH WALNUTS & ORANGE ZEST

walnuts, ¼ cup (1 oz/30 g) chopped
asparagus, 1½ lb (750 g)
olive oil, 1 Tbsp
orange zest, 1 Tbsp thin strips
sea salt, ⅛ tsp
MAKES 4 SERVINGS

1 Preheat oven to 350°F (180°C). Spread walnuts on a baking sheet and toast until lightly browned and fragrant, about 10 minutes. Immediately pour onto a plate to cool. Set aside. Increase oven temperature to 425°F (220°C).

2 Break off and discard tough stem ends from asparagus. Place spears in a baking dish. Sprinkle with olive oil, orange zest, and salt and toss to coat and mix well. Spread asparagus in a single layer.

3 Roast asparagus, stirring well once or twice, until tender when pierced with the tip of a sharp knife, about 10 minutes. Arrange on a platter, sprinkle with toasted walnuts, and serve right away.

High-heat roasting is a quick and healthy cooking technique that brings out the natural sugars in asparagus.

asparagus
- Rich in antioxidant and anti-inflammatory compounds
- Good source of fiber, iron, and folate
- Contains nutrients that support eye health

walnuts
- High in vitamin E
- Source of disease-fighting antioxidants
- Good source of fiber

per serving 110 calories, 5 g protein, 8 g carbs, 8 g fat (1 g saturated fat), 0 mg cholesterol, 4 g fiber, 70 mg sodium

In this sweet-and-tangy slaw, raw carrots develop flavor in a lemony dressing, and delicate Marcona almonds add a salty crunch. If you can't find Marconas, which are imported from Spain, feel free to use regular sliced almonds instead.

CARROT SLAW WITH LEMON–HONEY DRESSING

This no-cook side dish is a versatile addition to any meal. It is a good stand-in for classic coleslaw, which is typically made with high-fat mayonnaise.

carrots
- One of nature's richest sources of vitamin A and beta-carotene
- Good source of heart-healthy potassium
- Contain compounds that may fight cancer

fresh parsley
- Excellent source of vitamin K
- Contains compounds that promote eye health
- A natural breath freshener

per serving 240 calories, 4 g protein, 35 g carbs, 11 g fat (1.5 g saturated fat), 0 mg cholesterol, 6 g fiber, 270 mg sodium

extra-virgin olive oil, 2 Tbsp
sherry vinegar, 2 Tbsp
fresh lemon juice, 2 tsp
honey, 1½ tsp
sea salt, ¼ tsp
carrots, 1½ lb (750 g), peeled and grated
golden raisins, ½ cup (3 oz/90 g)
Marcona almonds, ¼ cup (1 oz/30 g)
fresh flat-leaf parsley, 1 Tbsp chopped

MAKES 4 SERVINGS

1 In a large salad bowl, whisk together olive oil, vinegar, lemon juice, honey, and salt.

2 Add carrots, raisins, almonds, and parsley to bowl and stir to mix and coat well. Serve right away, or cover and refrigerate for up to 1 day. Bring to room temperature before serving.

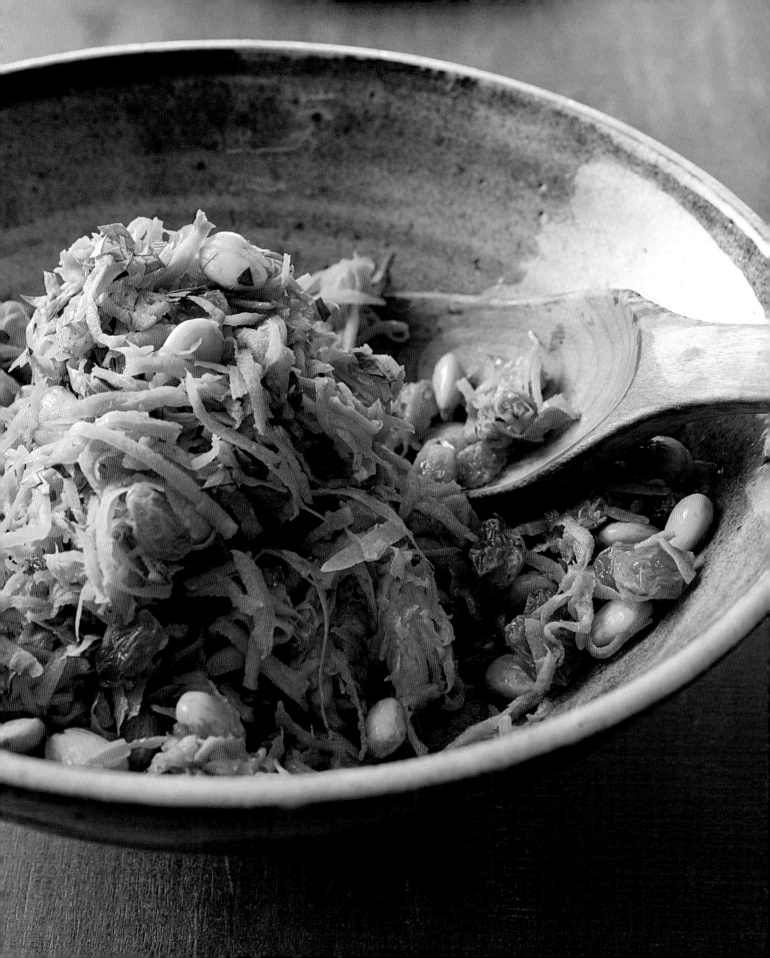

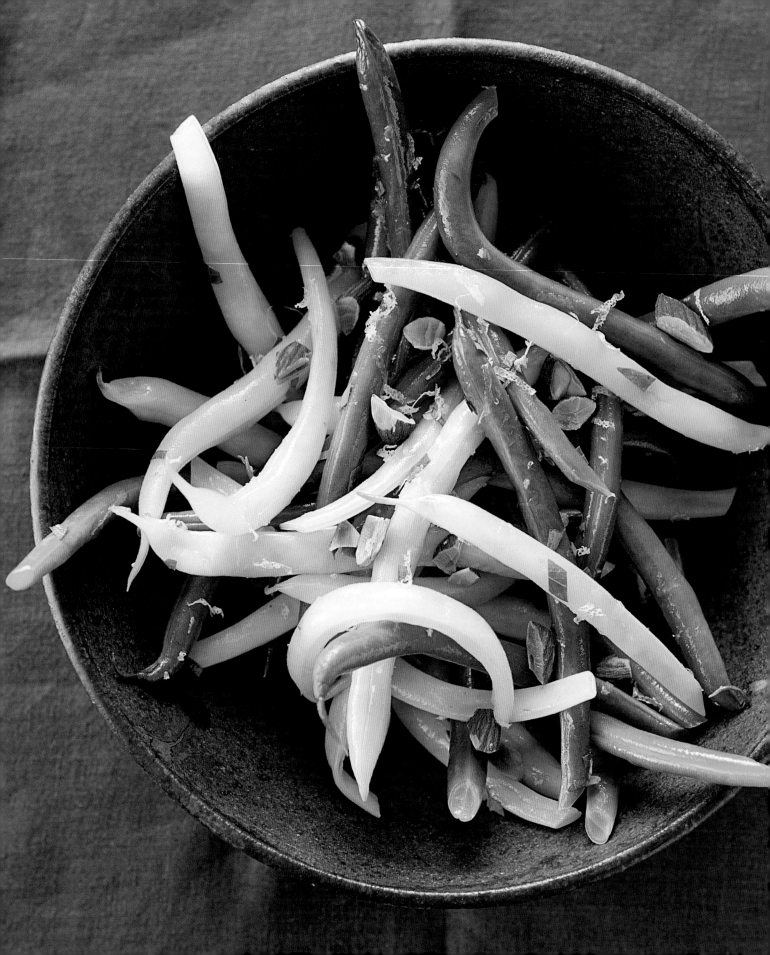

Celebrate summer's bounty with this colorful bean salad, a perfect companion to grilled meat or seafood and a welcome arrival at a barbecue or picnic table. You can blanch and marinate the beans in advance; top with the almonds just before serving.

SUMMER BEANS WITH LEMON & ALMONDS

whole almonds, ¼ cup (1½ oz/45 g)
green beans, ½ lb (250 g)
yellow wax beans, ½ lb (250 g)
extra-virgin olive oil, 1 Tbsp
fresh tarragon, 2 Tbsp chopped

grated zest and juice, from 1 lemon
sea salt, ¼ tsp
freshly ground pepper, to taste

MAKES 4 SERVINGS

1 Preheat oven to 350°F (180°C). Spread almonds on a baking sheet and toast until lightly browned and fragrant, about 10 minutes. Immediately pour onto a cutting board to cool, then chop coarsely. Set aside.

2 Trim beans and slice in half diagonally, if desired. Bring a large saucepan of lightly salted water to a boil and have ready a large bowl of ice water. Add beans to boiling water and cook just until tender, 3–4 minutes. Drain and transfer beans to ice water to cool. Drain well and put in a large bowl.

3 Add olive oil, tarragon, and lemon zest and juice to beans. Stir to mix well and season with salt and pepper. Set aside.

4 Transfer dressed beans to a platter, top with almonds, and serve right away.

Instead of butter, which is high in saturated fat, try tossing summer beans with a light vinaigrette made from olive oil and lemon juice. Note that salting the cooking water will increase the sodium content of the dish.

green beans
- Provide vitamins A, C, and K
- Good source of fiber
- Promotes heart, eye, and bone health

per serving 120 calories, 4 g protein, 11 g carbs, 8 g fat (1 g saturated fat), 0 mg cholesterol, 4 g fiber, 150 mg sodium

Try this approach with any hearty vegetable when you have leftover good-quality bread: slice it, toast it, and then whirl it in the food processor to make coarse fresh bread crumbs. You can also divide the mixture among heatproof ramekins to make individual servings.

KALE GRATIN WITH PARMESAN BREAD CRUMBS

Don't expect a creamy gratin bound with a cheesy sauce here—think of this kale-packed dish as a new way to serve hearty greens.

kale

- One of nature's top sources of zeaxanthin and lutein, nutrients linked to eye health
- Excellent source of vitamins A, C, and K
- Contains nutrients that help build strong bones

per serving 210 calories, 10 g protein, 22 g carbs, 11 g fat (2.5 g saturated fat), 5 mg cholesterol, 4 g fiber, 260 mg sodium

fresh whole-wheat sourdough bread crumbs, 1½ cups (3 oz/90 g) (see note)

Parmesan cheese, ½ cup (2 oz/60 g) freshly grated

olive oil, 3 Tbsp

garlic, 2 cloves, pressed or minced

kale, 2 lb (1 kg), stems and tough ribs removed, chopped

sea salt, ¼ tsp

MAKES 6 SERVINGS

1 Preheat oven to 375°F (190°C).

2 In a bowl, stir together bread crumbs, cheese, and 1 tablespoon of olive oil until well blended. Set aside.

3 Heat remaining 2 tablespoons olive oil in a large frying pan over medium heat. Add garlic and cook, stirring constantly, until fragrant but not browned, about 1 minute. Add kale and sprinkle with salt. Stir until kale is wilted and coated with oil. Add ¼ cup (2 fl oz/60 ml) water, cover, and steam until tender, 6–10 minutes, depending on age of kale. Transfer to a shallow gratin dish and smooth top. Sprinkle with bread-crumb mixture.

4 Bake until bread crumbs are golden brown, about 15 minutes. Let cool slightly, then serve right away.

This elegant, Japanese-inspired dish is a fast and delicious way to add greens to a meal. The spinach takes seconds to cook, and is easily shaped into little bundles for a unique presentation. Pack leftovers in an airtight container to add to your brown-bag lunch.

SESAME SPINACH SALAD

spinach, 1½ lb (750 g), stemmed and rinsed well
sake or dry white wine, ¼ cup (2 fl oz/60 ml)
low-sodium soy sauce, 2 Tbsp
sugar, 2 tsp
toasted sesame oil, 2 tsp
toasted sesame seeds, 2 Tbsp
MAKES 6 SERVINGS

1 Have ready a large bowl of ice water and place a colander in sink. Bring a pot of lightly salted water to a boil over high heat. Add half of spinach and cook just until wilted, about 1 minute. Using a slotted spoon, transfer spinach to ice water and stir gently to cool, then immediately lift out and transfer to colander to drain. Repeat process to cook, cool, and drain remaining spinach.

2 In another large bowl, whisk together sake, soy sauce, sugar, and sesame oil to make a dressing. Set aside.

3 Transfer cooled and drained spinach to a clean kitchen towel. Wrap tightly and squeeze or roll spinach to remove as much water as possible. Put in bowl with dressing and toss and stir to coat thoroughly.

4 Divide spinach into 6 portions and shape each into a cylindrical bundle, squeezing each tightly to compact the leaves. Arrange bundles on a serving plate. Spoon a little of the dressing left in the bowl over each. Sprinkle each bundle with about 1 teaspoon sesame seeds and serve right away.

Briefly cooking the spinach helps retain its nutrients. Note that salting the cooking water will increase the sodium content of the dish.

spinach
- Rich in vitamins A and K
- Provides small amounts of heart-healthy omega-3 fats
- Protects against cancer and promotes bone and eye health

sesame seeds
- Provide minerals such as iron, magnesium, and copper
- Linked to lowering cholesterol
- A surprising source of fiber

per serving 80 calories, 4 g protein, 7 g carbs, 3.5 g fat (0 g saturated fat), 0 mg cholesterol, 3 g fiber, 270 mg sodium

Here sweet green peas get a touch of tart luxury from a spoonful of crème fraîche. If you're lucky enough to find fresh pea tendrils (also called pea shoots), cut about 4 ounces (125 g) of them into short lengths, blanch them for about 1 minute, and stir them into the peas.

PEAS WITH MINT & PARMESAN

Peas can take longer to shell than to cook, but they're worth the trouble. Note that salting the cooking water will increase the dish's sodium content.

peas
- A legume providing plentiful vegetarian protein
- Contain a unique combination of protein and fiber that helps regulate blood sugar
- Rich source of vitamin C, folate, and B vitamins

fresh mint
- Soothes stomach ailments
- Essential oils contain antimicrobial properties
- May protect against cancer

per serving 90 calories, 6 g protein, 11 g carbs, 3 g fat (1.5 g saturated fat), 5 mg cholesterol, 4 g fiber, 240 mg sodium

crème fraîche, 2 Tbsp

fresh lemon juice, 1 tsp

sea salt, ¼ tsp

peas, 2 cups (10 oz/315 g), shelled from about 2 lb (1 kg) fresh peas in their pods, or frozen (not thawed)

fresh mint, 1 Tbsp coarsely chopped

Parmesan cheese, 1 oz (30 g), shaved with a vegetable peeler (about ¼ cup)

MAKES 4 SERVINGS

1 In a large bowl, whisk together crème fraîche, lemon juice, and salt.

2 Bring a saucepan of lightly salted water to a boil. If using fresh peas, add to boiling water and cook just until tender and bright green, about 3 minutes. If using frozen peas, add to boiling water and cook for 1 minute. Drain well.

3 Pour peas into bowl with crème fraîche mixture and add mint. Stir gently to combine and coat peas evenly. Garnish with Parmesan and serve right away.

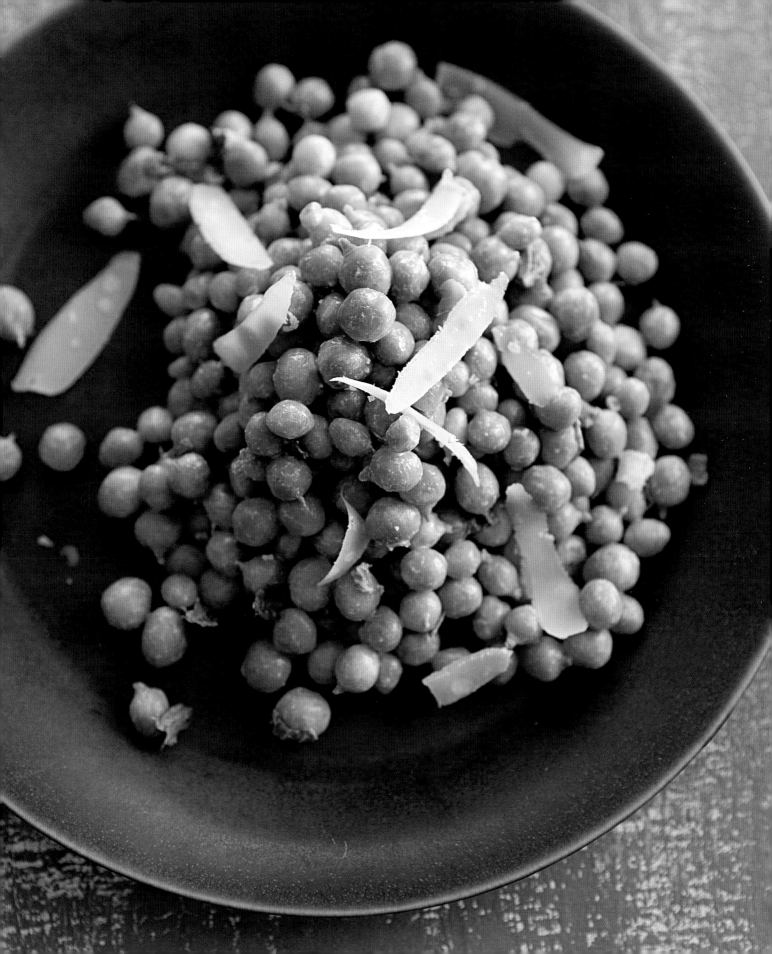

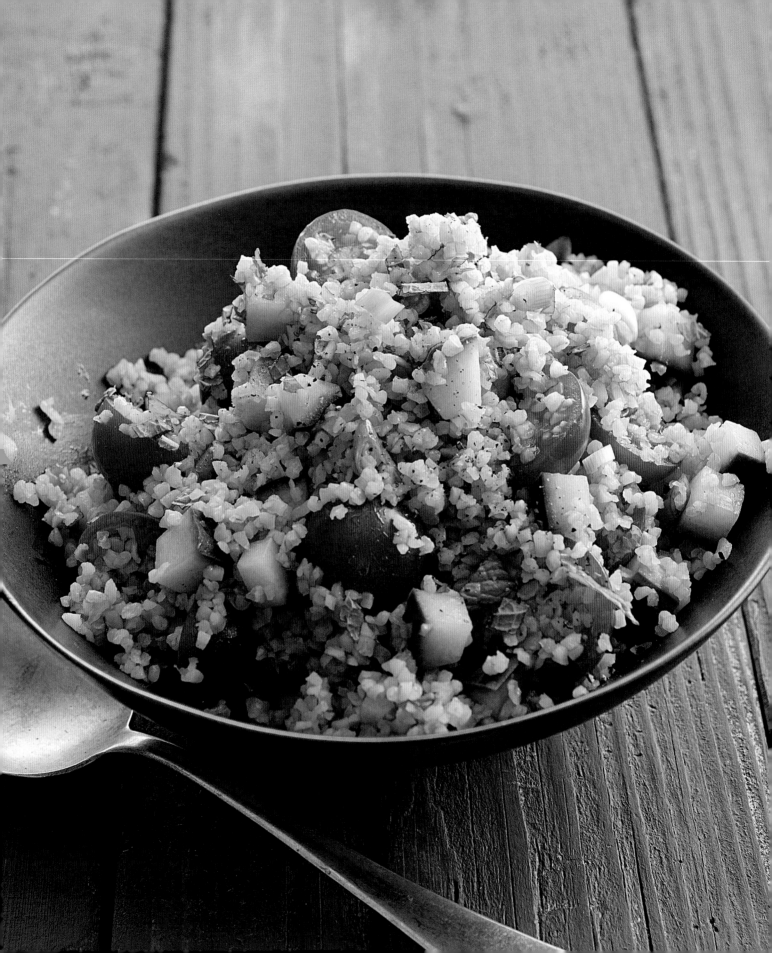

Bulgur is a sturdy, chewy form of wheat that readily soaks up juices and flavor from a dressing made with good olive oil and vinegar, sweet cherry tomatoes, and aromatic fresh mint. Serve it with grilled meat, or pack it along on your next picnic.

TABBOULEH WITH MINT & CHERRY TOMATOES

bulgur, 1 cup (6 oz/185 g)

cherry tomatoes, 2 cups (12 oz/375 g)

fresh lemon juice, 3 Tbsp

extra-virgin olive oil, 3 Tbsp

balsamic or red wine vinegar, 1 Tbsp

salt, ¼ tsp

freshly ground pepper

fresh mint leaves, ½ cup packed (½ oz/15 g), coarsely chopped

English cucumber, ½ cup (2½ oz/75 g) seeded and chopped

green onions, 3, white and pale green parts, thinly sliced

MAKES 4 SERVINGS

1 Put bulgur in a heatproof bowl. In a small saucepan, bring 1 cup (8 fl oz/ 250 ml) water to a boil. Pour water over bulgur, cover bowl tightly with aluminum foil, and let stand for 30 minutes.

2 Meanwhile, remove any stems from tomatoes and cut in half horizontally. In a large bowl, whisk together lemon juice, olive oil, vinegar, salt, and a few grindings of pepper to make a dressing.

3 Add tomatoes to bowl with dressing. Drain any remaining water from bulgur and add to tomato mixture along with mint, cucumber, and green onions. Taste and adjust seasoning and serve right away, or cover and refrigerate for up to 1 day. Bring to room temperature before serving.

Here's a great way to add more whole grains to your diet while taking advantage of fresh summer produce.

bulgur wheat
- Rich in insoluble fiber, which aids in digestion
- Packed with manganese, which helps support metabolism
- Excellent source of complex carbohydrates to regulate blood sugar

cucumbers
- Have been linked to a clear complexion
- Keep the skin on for extra nutrients

per serving 240 calories, 5 g protein, 33 g carbs, 11 g fat (1.5 g saturated fat), 0 mg cholesterol, 8 g fiber, 160 mg sodium

Tangy citrus, dried fruit, and toasted pine nuts flavor this savory Middle Eastern salad. Couscous, which, like pasta, is made from semolina, is available in many forms; choose the more nutritional whole-wheat version if available.

WHOLE-WHEAT COUSCOUS WITH GOLDEN RAISINS

Whole grains, healthful fats, fresh herbs, and fruit combine in this super-quick side dish. To reduce the fat content, omit the pine nuts.

whole-wheat couscous
- Plentiful in complex carbs and fiber to help keep you full
- Whole grains are slowly digested for sustained energy

raisins
- Excellent source of potassium for healthy blood pressure
- Contain antioxidants and fiber
- Add natural sweetness to foods

per serving 370 calories, 10 g protein, 62 g carbs, 10 g fat (1 g saturated fat), 0 mg cholesterol, 4 g fiber, 300 mg sodium

orange, 1
saffron threads, ⅛ tsp
pine nuts, ¼ cup (1 oz/30 g)
olive oil, 1 Tbsp
whole-wheat couscous, 1½ cups (9 oz/280 g)
golden raisins, ¼ cup (1½ oz/45 g)

salt, ½ tsp
ground cinnamon, ¼ tsp
fresh mint leaves, ½ cup (½ oz/15 g), chopped
fresh lemon juice, ¼ cup (2 fl oz/60 ml)
freshly ground pepper, to taste

MAKES 4 SERVINGS

1 Remove 1 teaspoon finely grated zest from orange. Juice orange and measure out ¼ cup (2 fl oz/60 ml) juice. (Save any extra juice for another use, or drink it.) Set zest and juice aside.

2 Put saffron threads in a small, dry frying pan over medium heat and toast, shaking pan constantly, until fragrant and a shade darker, about 1 minute. Immediately transfer to a small bowl and let cool, then crumble with your fingertips. Set aside. In the same frying pan over medium heat, toast pine nuts, stirring constantly, until lightly browned and fragrant, 3–5 minutes. Immediately pour onto a plate to cool. Set aside.

3 In a large heatproof bowl, drizzle olive oil over couscous and stir to coat well. Scatter raisins on top.

4 In a small saucepan, bring 2 cups (16 fl oz/500 ml) water to a boil. Stir in saffron, salt, and cinnamon and pour over couscous. Cover bowl tightly with aluminum foil and let stand until couscous is tender and liquid is absorbed, about 5 minutes.

5 Remove foil and fluff couscous with a fork to separate grains. Stir in mint, pine nuts, orange zest, orange juice, and lemon juice. Season with pepper and serve.

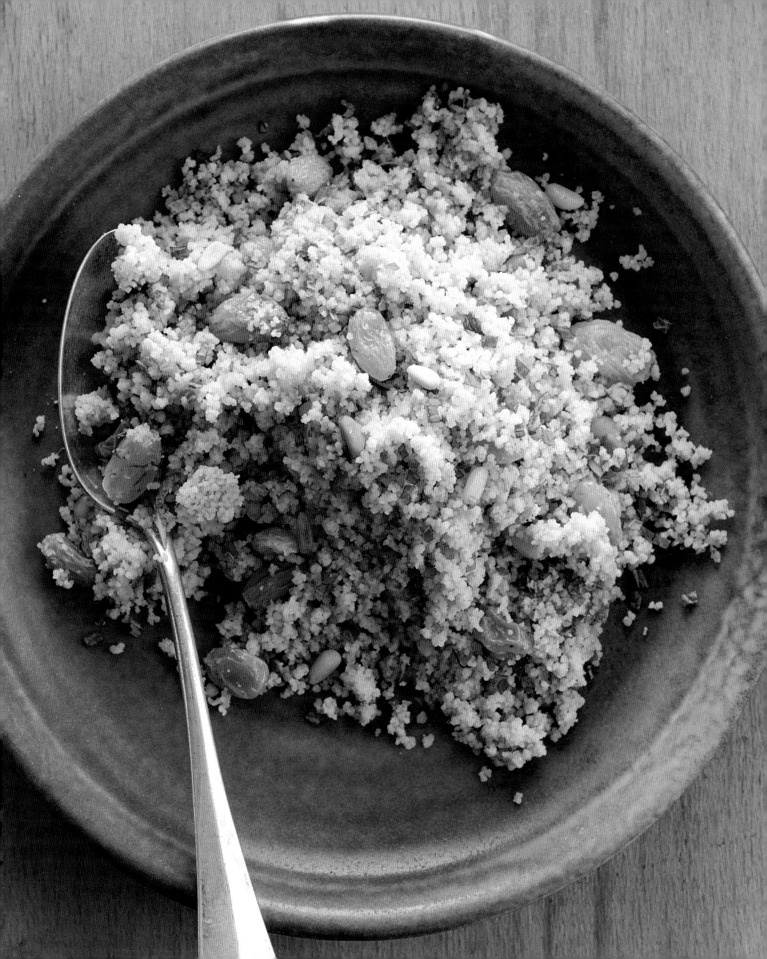

This orange-scented pilaf makes a light meatless meal or a nice accompaniment to grilled or roasted meats. A powerhouse of nutrition, quinoa is great to keep on hand in the pantry for a quick, whole-grain side dish.

QUINOA PILAF WITH APRICOTS & ALMONDS

fresh orange juice, ½ cup
(4 fl oz/125 ml)

ground turmeric, ⅛ tsp

salt, ⅛ tsp plus ¼ tsp

quinoa, 1 cup (8 oz/250 g)

slivered almonds, ⅓ cup (2 oz/60 g)

dried apricots, ⅓ cup (2 oz/60 g),
thinly sliced

extra-virgin olive oil, 1 Tbsp

fresh lemon juice, 1 Tbsp

minced orange zest, from 1 orange

freshly ground pepper, to taste

MAKES 4 SERVINGS

You can cut down on the fat in the dish by omitting the almonds and substituting 3 or 4 thinly sliced green onions.

quinoa
- Good source of complete protein and fiber
- Rich in minerals such as iron, manganese, and phosphorus
- Excellent choice for people on a gluten-free eating plan

turmeric
- Linked to brain function and heart health
- Possesses potent anti-inflammatory properties
- May help prevent cancer

per serving 280 calories, 9 g protein, 40 g carbs, 11 g fat (1 g saturated fat), 0 mg cholesterol, 5 g fiber, 200 mg sodium

1 In a saucepan, combine orange juice, turmeric, ⅛ teaspoon salt, and 1 cup (8 fl oz/250 ml) water. Bring to a boil over high heat.

2 Put quinoa in a fine-mesh strainer and rinse under cold running water. Add quinoa to pan, cover, reduce heat to maintain a gentle simmer, and cook until liquid is absorbed, about 20 minutes.

3 Meanwhile, preheat oven to 350°F (180°C). Spread almonds on a baking sheet and toast until lightly browned and fragrant, about 10 minutes. Immediately pour onto a plate to cool.

4 Fluff quinoa with a fork to separate grains and stir in almonds, apricots, olive oil, lemon juice, and orange zest. Season with ¼ teaspoon salt and pepper. Serve right away.

Serve these beans alongside Mexican-inspired meals, such as scrambled egg *chilaquiles* (page 51), steak fajitas (page 142), or salmon tacos (page 132), or spoon them into burritos. You can use black beans you've cooked yourself, or good-quality canned beans.

CREAMY REFRIED BLACK BEANS

olive oil, 1 Tbsp

yellow onion, ¼ cup (1½ oz/45 g) minced

mild green chiles such as pasilla, 2 Tbsp seeded and minced

garlic, 1 clove, pressed or minced

low-sodium cooked black beans, 3 cups (21 oz/655 g), cooking or canning liquid reserved

ground cumin, ½ tsp

chili powder, ½ tsp

sea salt, ¼ tsp

fresh lime juice, 1–2 Tbsp

MAKES 6 SERVINGS

1 Heat olive oil in a saucepan over medium heat. Add onion, chiles, and garlic and sauté, reducing heat as necessary to prevent scorching, until onion and chiles are soft and wilted, 5–8 minutes.

2 Transfer onion mixture to a food processor. (Reserve pan.) Add beans, cumin, chili powder, salt, and 2 tablespoons reserved bean cooking liquid or juices from can, or water. Whirl until mixture is a smooth purée, adding up to 2 tablespoons more liquid if necessary to achieve desired consistency.

3 Return bean mixture to pan. Place over low heat and stir until hot. Stir in 1 tablespoon lime juice and remove from heat. Taste and adjust seasoning with additional lime juice, if needed. Serve right away, or store in an airtight container in the refrigerator for up to 3 days.

Refried beans are traditionally cooked in lard, but this modern take on a favorite Mexican dish uses heart-healthy, fruity olive oil instead.

black beans
- Rich source of potent anti-inflammatories
- Excellent source of vegetable protein and fiber
- Legumes are slowly digested to promote fullness

onions
- Linked to lower cancer risk
- Cutting onions 5–10 minutes before using releases more of their health-promoting compounds

per serving 140 calories, 8 g protein, 22 g carbs, 3 g fat (0 g saturated fat), 0 mg cholesterol, 8 g fiber, 105 mg sodium

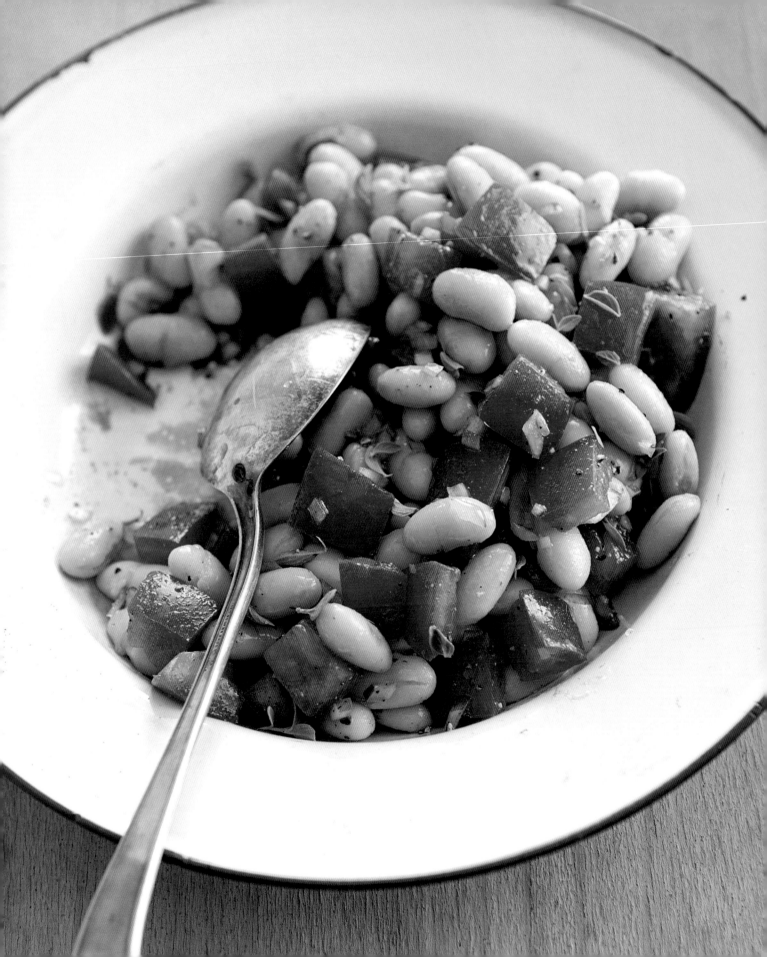

This humble side dish relies on top-notch ingredients, so use good-quality canned beans (or better yet, start with dried and cook your own, page 155), ripe tomatoes, fruity olive oil, and fresh herbs. Basil, parsley, or sage can be substituted for the oregano.

WHITE BEANS WITH TOMATOES & OREGANO

red onion, ¼ cup (1¼ oz/37 g) finely chopped

low-sodium cannellini or other white beans, 2 cans (15 oz/470 g each)

ripe tomatoes, 2

balsamic vinegar, 2 Tbsp

extra-virgin olive oil, 1 Tbsp

fresh oregano leaves, 2 Tbsp

sea salt, ¼ tsp

freshly ground pepper, to taste

MAKES 4 SERVINGS

1 Put onion in a fine-mesh strainer and rinse under cold running water. Drain well. Put beans in a colander, drain, rinse well, and drain again.

2 Cut tomatoes in half horizontally. Gently squeeze out seeds, using your fingertip to nudge them if necessary. Chop coarsely. You should have about 1½ cups (9 oz/280 g).

3 In a bowl, mix beans, tomatoes, vinegar, olive oil, oregano, onion, salt, and pepper. Serve right away, or cover and refrigerate for up to 4 hours. Bring to room temperature before serving.

Three staples of the famed heart-healthy Mediterranean diet star in this easy side dish.

white beans
- Loaded with heart-smart fiber, folate, and potassium
- Help stabilize blood sugar
- Rinsing canned beans can lower their sodium by 40 percent

fresh oregano
- Has antibacterial properties
- Packed with powerful antioxidants
- Contains nutrients linked to bone and heart health

per serving 290 calories, 16 g protein, 50 g carbs, 4 g fat (.5 g saturated fat), 0 mg cholesterol, 11 g fiber, 160 mg sodium

This tiny, quick-cooking member of the legume family has a nutty, peppery flavor and a firm texture that holds up well to marinating. Pair this side dish with a simple main course, like panfried turkey sausages, rotisserie chicken, or poached salmon.

LENTILS WITH RED PEPPERS & SHALLOTS

small green or brown lentils, 1 cup (7 oz/220 g)

extra-virgin olive oil, 2 Tbsp

shallots, 4–6, thinly sliced

roasted red bell peppers, ½ cup (3 oz/90 g), jarred or homemade (page 214), drained and cut into strips

sherry vinegar, 3 Tbsp, plus more if needed

fresh flat-leaf parsley, 3 Tbsp chopped

sea salt, ½ tsp

MAKES 4 SERVINGS

Lentils are a good option when you want to include legumes in a meal, but didn't plan ahead for an overnight soak.

lentils
- Outstanding source of heart-smart folate, fiber, and potassium
- Provide lean vegetable protein
- Cook quickly

shallots
- Rich in compounds that prevent cancer and heart disease
- Possess potent anti-inflammatory properties
- Milder in aroma and flavor than onions

per serving 300 calories, 14 g protein, 41 g carbs, 10 g fat (1.5 g saturated fat), 0 mg cholesterol, 15 g fiber, 310 mg sodium

1 Pick over lentils for stones or grit. Rinse in a colander and drain thoroughly.

2 Bring a pot of water to a boil over high heat. Add lentils, reduce heat to low, and simmer until lentils are tender to the bite, 18–25 minutes.

3 While lentils are cooking, heat 1 tablespoon of olive oil in large nonstick frying pan over medium-high heat. Add shallots and cook until softened, 2–3 minutes. Reduce heat to medium-low and cook, stirring often, until shallots have caramelized to a nice golden brown, 5–8 minutes longer. Remove from heat and set aside.

4 Drain lentils and transfer to a bowl. Stir in peppers, vinegar, parsley, salt, shallots, and remaining 1 tablespoon olive oil. Taste and adjust seasoning with vinegar, if needed.

5 Serve warm or at room temperature, stirring well once more before serving.

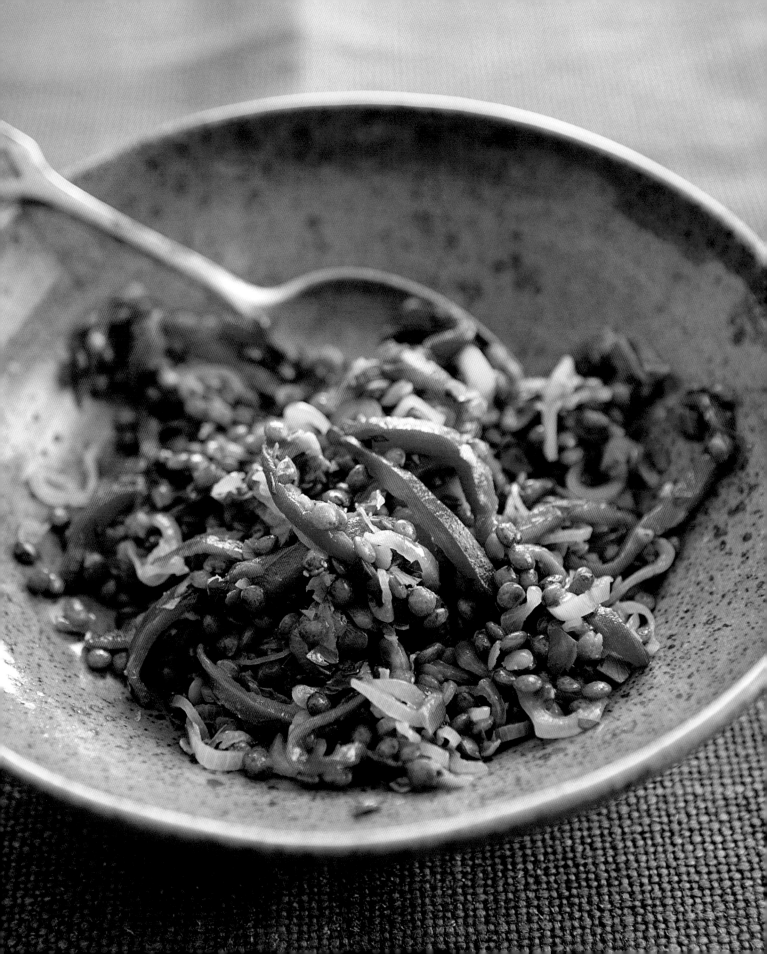

Sweet endings are the ultimate finish to a memorable meal. Choose light and fruity desserts to balance out an indulgent meal, or treat yourself to something rich and decadent if you've eaten lightly.

DESSERT

QUICK-FIX IDEAS FOR DESSERT

COOK IT IN A FLASH

CHOCOLATE-DIPPED BANANAS Line a baking sheet with parchment paper. Chop dark chocolate into small pieces and place in a double boiler or a heatproof bowl set over but not touching a pan of barely simmering water. Melt the chocolate, stirring occasionally, just until smooth. Slice a few bananas into 1-inch (2.5-cm) rounds and drop them, one at a time, into the melted chocolate. Lift each slice out with a fork and place on the baking sheet. Sprinkle with chopped nuts, if you like. Refrigerate or freeze until ready to serve.

BLUEBERRY SAUCE Simmer 1 pint (8 oz/250 g) blueberries in a small saucepan with 2 tablespoons water and honey to taste until soft. Mix 1 teaspoon cornstarch with a splash of orange juice in a small bowl. Add the cornstarch mixture to the simmering fruit and stir until slightly thickened. Serve over low-fat or nonfat frozen yogurt or another dessert.

CARAMELIZED APPLES Sauté sliced apples or pears in a saucepan with a small amount of butter and brown sugar until the slices begin to turn brown and caramelize. Mix in a handful of toasted hazelnuts or walnuts. Serve over thin buckwheat crêpes, or with a dollop of thick yogurt.

NO COOKING NEEDED

BALSAMIC STRAWBERRIES Choose an aged balsamic vinegar and the ripest strawberries you can find. Halve the strawberries, drizzle them with a little balsamic, and sprinkle with freshly ground pepper.

COOKIE "TARTLETS" Spread thin, crisp gingersnaps or your favorite small, flat cookies with purchased marmalade or fruit jam. Arrange fresh blueberries or raspberries on top. Or, for ice-cream sandwiches, spread slightly softened nonfat frozen yogurt between the cookies and freeze until firm.

MANGO-PINEAPPLE SAUCE Put the peeled flesh of 2 ripe mangoes in a blender. Add a little minced fresh ginger, a splash of maple syrup, and a cupful of pineapple juice. Purée until smooth. Serve over tapioca or slices of angel food cake.

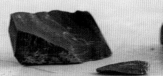

MAKE IT AHEAD

FROZEN BERRY YOGURT Whirl together frozen blackberries, blueberries, or raspberries in a food processor or blender, with a squeeze of lemon juice. Add cold low-fat or nonfat yogurt and whirl again until blended. If desired, sweeten with a little honey, maple syrup, or agave nectar. Transfer to a covered container and freeze until ready to serve.

DARK CHOCOLATE BARK Combine melted bittersweet chocolate with dried fruit and nuts for an impressive dessert that comes together in minutes. Follow the recipe for Dark Chocolate–Blueberry Bark (page 207), swapping in the mix-ins of your choice.

JUICE POPS With fresh fruit juice and an ice pop mold, you can create all kinds of healthy frozen treats ready to eat at a moment's notice. Try Pomegranate-Tangerine Ice Pops (page 191) or create your own flavor combinations using your favorite all-natural juices, like raspberry-lemon, pineapple-orange, or cherry-lime.

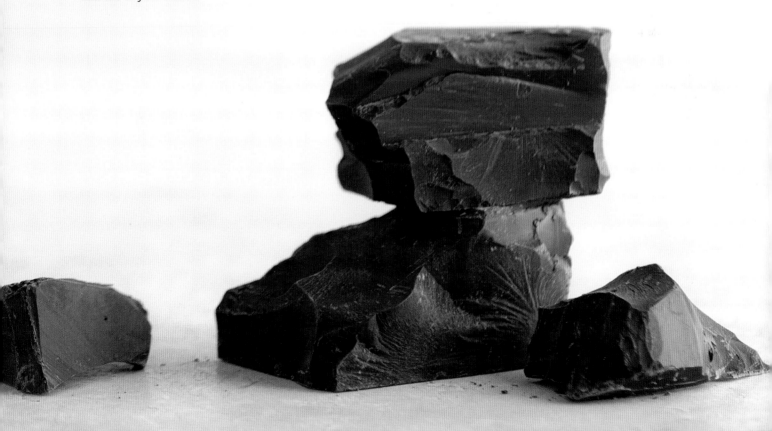

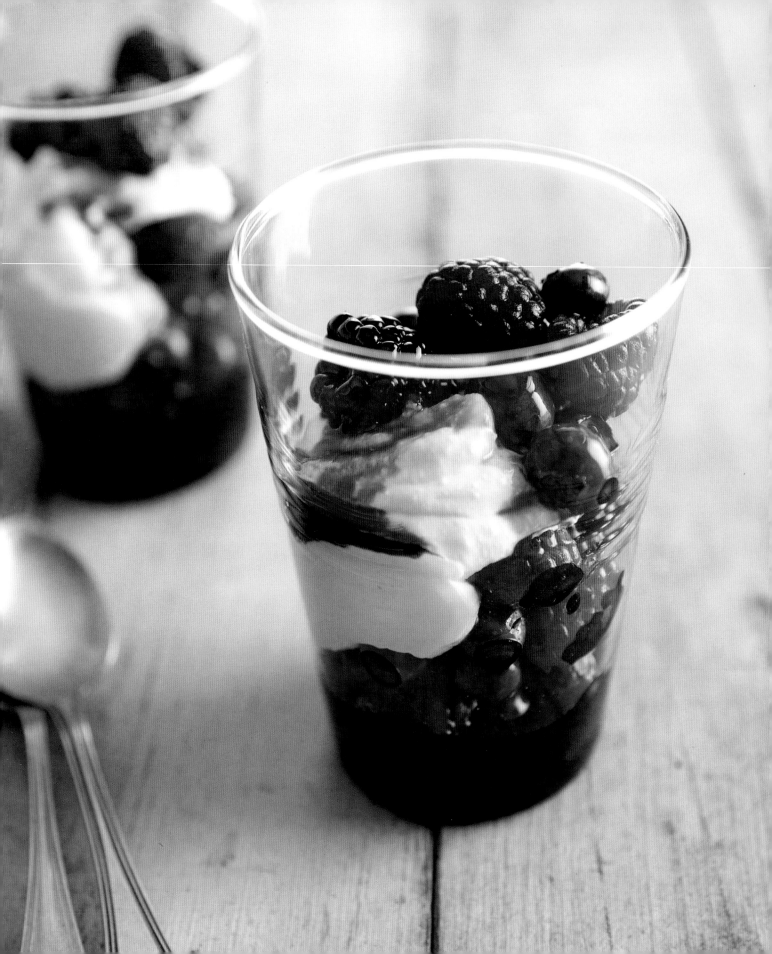

Berries are elevated to a heady level in this elegant, and adult-only, dessert that is light and healthy with a touch of richness. You can prepare the red wine syrup and ricotta mixture in advance and assemble the components just before serving.

WINE-SPIKED BERRIES WITH RICOTTA

orange, 1 large

dry red wine, 1½ cups (12 fl oz/375 ml)

sugar, ½ cup (4 oz/125 g) plus 2 Tbsp

mixed raspberries, blueberries, and/or blackberries, 2 cups (8 oz/250 g)

part-skim ricotta cheese, 1 cup (8 oz/250 g)

Grand Marnier liqueur, 1 Tbsp

pure vanilla extract, ¼ tsp

MAKES 4 SERVINGS

1 Using a sharp paring knife, cut two 2–3-inch (5–7.5-cm) strips of zest from orange. Using fine rasps of a handheld grater or a microplane, remove 1 teaspoon finely grated zest from another section of orange. Set both zests aside (save orange for another use).

2 In a small saucepan over medium-high heat, combine wine, ½ cup sugar, and zest strips and cook, stirring constantly, until sugar dissolves, about 3 minutes. Bring to a boil, then reduce heat to medium and simmer until liquid is reduced by about one-third, 10–15 minutes. Remove from heat and let cool.

3 Put berries in a bowl. Remove zest strips from syrup and pour over berries.

4 In a food processor, combine ricotta, liqueur, vanilla, grated orange zest, and 2 tablespoons sugar and process until smooth. Spoon berries with some syrup into glasses or small bowls and top with a dollop of ricotta mixture. Serve right away.

Fresh berries marinated in syrup make a tempting addition to after-dinner parfaits. For an even lower-fat version of this dessert, substitute plain nonfat yogurt for the ricotta.

part-skim ricotta cheese
- Rich in whey protein, which is linked to weight control
- Good source of nutrients linked to bone health and blood pressure control
- Contains more than four times the calcium of cottage cheese

per serving 330 calories, 8 g protein, 45 g carbs, 5 g fat (3 g saturated fat), 20 mg cholesterol, 5 g fiber, 80 mg sodium

Use either fresh or frozen blackberries in this recipe. If using frozen, buy ones without added sugar, and thaw them before using, reserving the juice. Make sure you have an ice-cream maker and enough time to let the mixture freeze into a tangy, irresistible treat.

BLACKBERRY—BUTTERMILK SHERBET

This buttermilk-based sherbet tastes like decadent ice cream, but is a lot lower in fat, and gets an antioxidant boost from the blackberries.

blackberries
- Richer in antioxidants than most other berries
- Outstanding source of fiber
- Contain compounds that fight cancer and improve short-term memory

buttermilk
- Excellent source of calcium for strong bones
- Rich source of potassium
- Naturally low in fat

per serving 110 calories, 3 g protein, 25 g carbs, .5 g fat (0 g saturated fat), 0 mg cholesterol, 3 g fiber, 55 mg sodium

blackberries, 2½ cups (10 oz/315 g)

sugar, ½ cup (4 oz/125 g)

low-fat (1%) buttermilk, 1¼ cups (10 fl oz/310 ml)

fresh lemon juice, 2 tsp

MAKES ABOUT 1½ PINTS (24 OZ/750 G); 6 SERVINGS

1 In a blender or food processor, whirl blackberries (along with any juices from thawed frozen berries) until smooth. Pour purée into fine-mesh strainer set over bowl, pressing on solids to extract as much purée as possible (you should have about 1 cup/8 fl oz/250 ml purée). Discard solids.

2 Add sugar and whisk until dissolved. Whisk in buttermilk and lemon juice.

3 Freeze mixture in an ice-cream maker according to manufacturer's instructions. Transfer to an airtight container and freeze until firm enough to scoop, 4–6 hours.

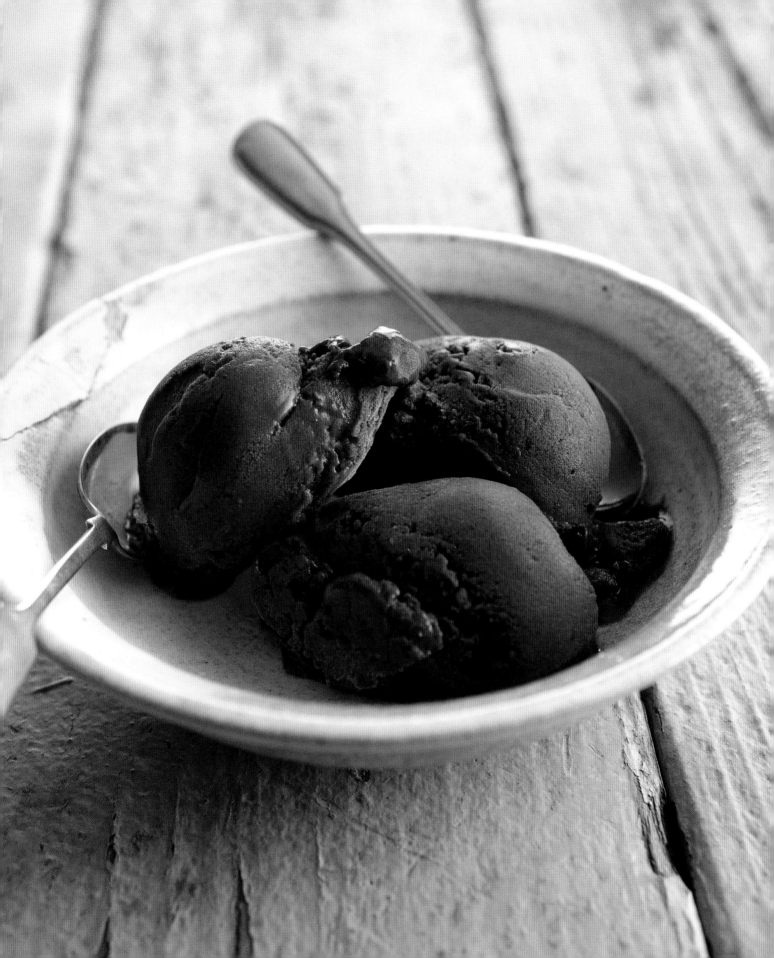

Here, sweet, seedless watermelon is puréed and frozen for the ultimate summer dessert. Other types of summer melons, such as cantaloupe or honeydew, would work here as well; taste and adjust the amounts of sugar and lime juice before freezing.

WATERMELON—LIME GRANITA

This nonfat icy treat, an elegant twist on watermelon wedges with lime, is sure to become a summertime favorite.

watermelon
- One of nature's richest sources of lycopene, shown to prevent some types of cancer
- Excellent source of vitamin C
- Rich in amino acids that detoxify the blood

fresh herbs
- Nearly calorie-free way to boost flavor
- Have antibacterial and anti-inflammatory properties

per serving 90 calories, 1 g protein, 24 g carbs, 0 g fat (0 g saturated fat), 0 mg cholesterol, 1 g fiber, 2.5 mg sodium

seedless watermelon, 3 lb (1.5 kg), peeled and cut into 1-inch (2.5-cm) cubes (about 4½ cups/20 oz/625 g)

sugar, 3 Tbsp

fresh lime juice, 3 Tbsp

slivered fresh mint or basil leaves, for garnish

MAKES 6 SERVINGS

1 In a blender, whirl watermelon, sugar, and lime juice until very smooth. Pour into a large shallow bowl.

2 Place bowl in freezer. Stir mixture about every hour, breaking up any ice crystals with a fork, until mixture is granular and slushy, 4–6 hours. Cover and freeze for up to 1 day, or spoon into tall glasses, top with a few slivers of mint, and serve at once.

Fresh pomegranate juice is available in the refrigerated juice section of most supermarkets. Its sweet, tart flavor is suited to a simple preparation like these vibrant, refreshing pops. Ice pop molds are easy to find and worth having around for easy warm-weather treats.

POMEGRANATE-TANGERINE ICE POPS

pomegranate juice, 2 cups
(16 fl oz/500 ml)

fresh tangerine or orange juice, ⅔ cup
(5 fl oz/160 ml)

sugar, 3 Tbsp

MAKES 6 POPS

1 In a large bowl, whisk together pomegranate juice, tangerine juice, and sugar until sugar is completely dissolved, about 2 minutes.

2 Ladle mixture into ice pop molds. Attach cover and insert sticks. Place molds in freezer and freeze until firm, at least 6 hours and up to 2 weeks.

3 To serve, run hot water over outsides of mold (below rim) for a few seconds, then gently tug on sticks to remove.

Packed with vitamins but not a bit of fat, these juice pops are as healthy as they are fun to eat.

pomegranates
- Excellent source of antioxidants
- Linked to cardiovascular health
- Good source of vitamin C and fiber

tangerines
- Rich in antioxidants that protect against cancer
- Packed with vitamin C
- Good source of fiber

per pop 90 calories,
0 g protein, 22 g carbs,
0 g fat (0 g saturated fat),
0 mg cholesterol, 0 g fiber,
3.5 mg sodium

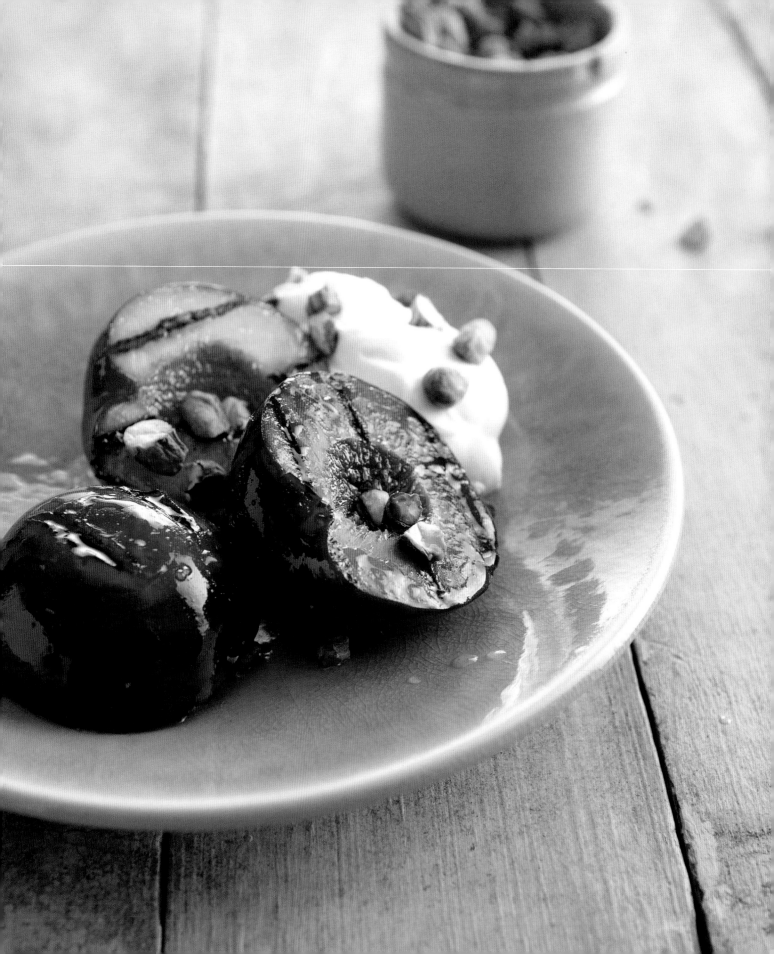

Thick, tart Greek yogurt makes a rich topping for this simple fruit dessert that is gorgeous on the plate and a perfect end for a summer barbecue. Any stone fruit, such as nectarines or pluots, can be used in place of the plums; increase the cooking time slightly for larger fruits.

GRILLED PLUMS WITH PISTACHIOS & YOGURT

canola oil, 1 Tbsp

firm-ripe plums such as Santa Rosa, 6, halved and pitted

raw or turbinado sugar, 2 Tbsp

plain low-fat Greek yogurt, 1 cup (8 oz/250 g)

pistachios, ¼ cup (1 oz/30 g), chopped

MAKES 4 SERVINGS

1 Build a hot fire in a charcoal grill or preheat a gas grill to high. Brush grill rack with canola oil.

2 Place plum halves, cut side down, directly over heat; close lid if using a gas grill. Cook until flesh is soft and lightly grill-marked, 1–2 minutes.

3 Using a metal spatula or tongs, carefully turn plums over and sprinkle cut sides with sugar. Continue to cook until sugar is melted and plums are tender but still hold their shape, about 3 minutes longer.

4 Transfer plums to dessert plates or shallow bowls, placing 3 halves on each. Stir yogurt well and spoon a dollop alongside; sprinkle with pistachios. Serve right away.

If you like yogurt parfaits for breakfast, you will love this version that's been reconfigured into a healthy dessert.

plums
- Good source of fiber
- Loaded with vitamin C and antioxidants
- Provide potassium for strong bones and healthy blood pressure

pistachios
- Rich in vitamin E needed for a healthy immune system
- Nuts are a good source of vegetarian protein
- Provide heart-smart potassium, monounsaturated fat, and fiber

per serving 180 calories, 8 g protein, 20 g carbs, 8 g fat (1 g saturated fat), 0 mg cholesterol, 2 g fiber, 25 mg sodium

You can make an extra batch of this easy crisp topping and freeze it in a zippered plastic bag for several months. That way, you're ready at a moment's notice to bake up a great fruit dessert. In the summertime, swap in plums and blueberries, or peaches and blackberries.

APPLE-CRANBERRY CRISP

These two cool-weather fruits top the nutritional charts, and the oat-and-nut topping delivers even more antioxidant power.

apples
- Rich in quercetin, a plant compound linked to cancer prevention
- Contain nutrients that regulate blood sugar
- Linked to weight loss

cranberries
- Rich source of protective phytochemicals
- Improve digestive function and liver health
- Contain nutrients that work to enhance heart health

per serving 350 calories, 5 g protein, 56 g carbs, 13 g fat (6 g saturated fat), 25 mg cholesterol, 4 g fiber, 65 mg sodium

rolled oats, 1 cup (3 oz/90 g)

all-purpose flour, ¾ cup (3 oz/90 g)

light brown sugar, ½ cup (3½ oz/105 g) firmly packed

ground cinnamon, ¾ tsp

salt, ¼ tsp

unsalted butter, ½ cup (4 oz/125 g), cut into pieces

walnuts, ⅓ cup (1⅓ oz/40 g) chopped

granulated sugar, ⅓ cup (3 oz/90 g)

cornstarch, 1 Tbsp

apples, 3 lb (1.5 kg), peeled, cored, and sliced

fresh or frozen cranberries, 1 cup (4 oz/125 g)

MAKES 10 SERVINGS

1 Preheat oven to 375°F (190°C).

2 In a bowl, combine oats, flour, brown sugar, cinnamon, and salt and stir to mix well. Scatter in butter pieces. Using an electric mixer fitted with paddle attachment on low speed, or with your fingertips, mix or rub in butter until uniform coarse crumbs form and mixture begins to come together. Stir in chopped walnuts.

3 In a large bowl, whisk together granulated sugar and cornstarch until well blended. Add apples and cranberries and toss to coat and mix well. Pour fruit into a 9-inch (23-cm) square or round baking dish. Sprinkle evenly with oat mixture.

4 Bake until topping is golden brown and apples are tender when pierced with a knife, 50–60 minutes. Transfer to a wire rack and let crisp rest for at least 15 minutes before serving. Serve warm or at room temperature.

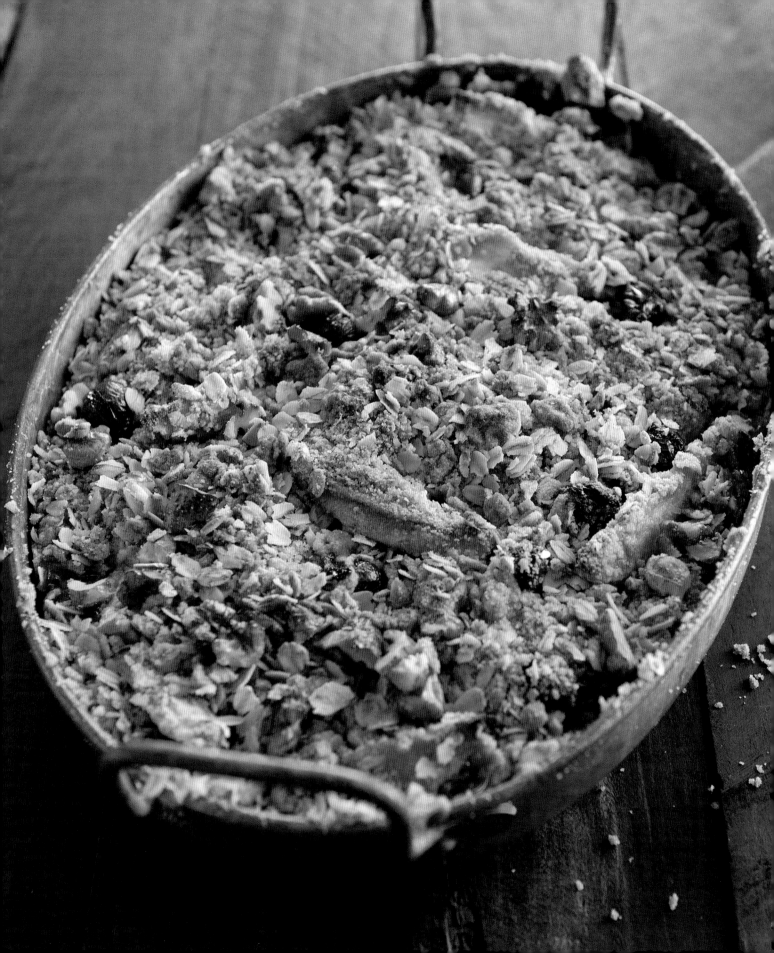

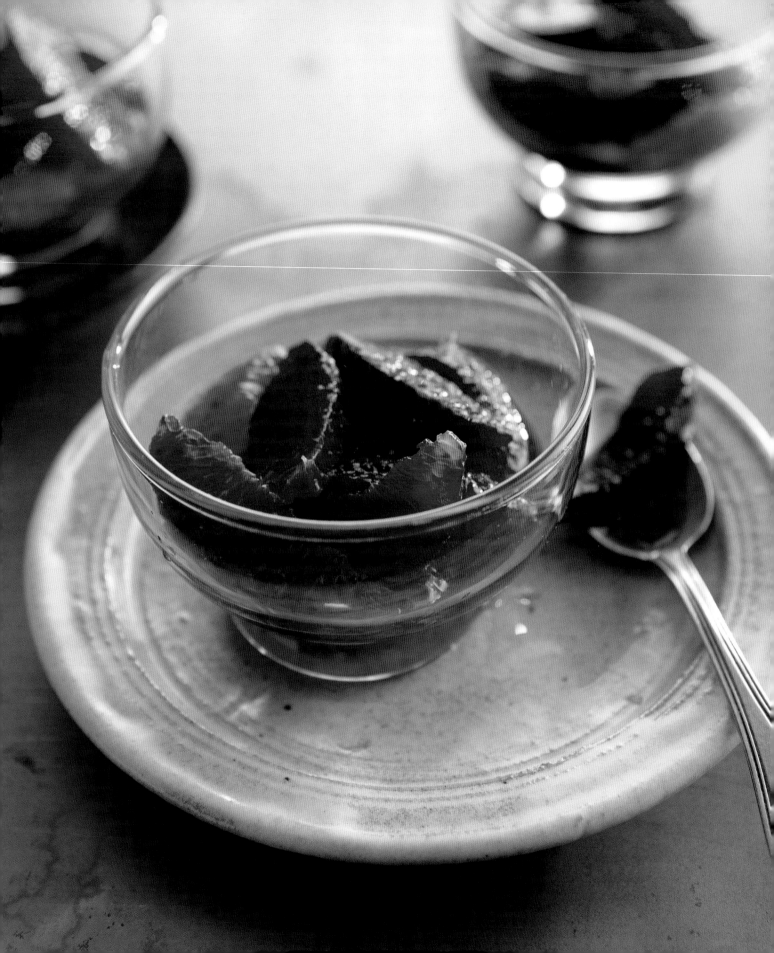

When you see blood oranges in the produce aisle or at your local farmers' market, buy a big bag and take the opportunity to turn them into eye-catching dishes like this super-simple dessert. Segmenting the fruit takes a little practice, but it makes a nice presentation.

MARINATED BLOOD ORANGES

blood or navel oranges, 3 lb (1.5 kg)

fresh lemon juice, 1 Tbsp

sugar, 2 Tbsp

orange liqueur such as Tuaca or Grand Marnier, ⅓ cup (3 fl oz/80 ml)

MAKES 6 SERVINGS

1 Using a sharp knife, cut a thin slice off both ends of each orange, then cut away peel and bitter white pith, following fruit's curve. Holding fruit over a bowl, cut on either side of each segment to free it from the membrane, letting segments and juices fall into bowl.

2 In a small bowl, stir together lemon juice, sugar, and orange liqueur. Pour mixture over orange segments and toss gently to combine. Cover and refrigerate until well chilled, at least 3 hours or up to 24 hours.

3 Spoon fruit and syrup into small bowls or glasses and serve right away.

This dish proves that dessert doesn't have to be a decadent, complicated affair; sometimes showcasing a single seasonal fruit is the best finale to a meal.

blood oranges
- Rich in compounds that help fight cancer
- Excellent source of vitamin C for a strong immune system
- Ample amounts of potassium and fiber support heart health

per serving 170 calories, 2 g protein, 38 g carbs, 0 g fat (0 g saturated fat), 0 mg cholesterol, 5 g fiber, 1.5 mg sodium

Creamy and slightly tart, this fresh-tasting dessert gets extra tang from seasonal berries tossed with brown sugar and a few drops of balsamic vinegar. It comes together quickly, but needs at least 8 hours to set, so make it a day or two before you plan to serve it.

YOGURT PANNA COTTA WITH BALSAMIC BERRIES

Panna cotta is often made with heavy cream; this version uses low-fat milk and yogurt for a much healthier, and still delicious, spin on the classic.

low-fat yogurt
- Quick, convenient source of calcium and protein
- Linked to digestive and immune system health
- Look for "live and active cultures" on the label

strawberries
- Loaded with vitamin C
- Rich in cancer-preventing compounds
- May have anti-aging effects on the brain

per serving 210 calories,
11 g protein, 34 g carbs, 4 g fat (1.5 g saturated fat), 10 mg cholesterol, 2 g fiber, 105 mg sodium

unflavored gelatin, 2 tsp (one 1-oz/30-g envelope)

low-fat (2%) milk, 1½ cups (12 fl oz/375 ml)

vanilla bean, 1, split lengthwise, or 1 tsp vanilla extract

granulated sugar, ½ cup (4 oz/125 g)

plain low-fat yogurt, 2 cups (16 oz/500 g)

canola oil, 2 tsp

mixed fresh berries such as blackberries, raspberries, and sliced strawberries, 1¼ cups (5 oz/155 g)

light brown sugar, 2 Tbsp firmly packed

balsamic vinegar, 2 tsp

MAKES 6 SERVINGS

1 In a small bowl, sprinkle gelatin over ½ cup (4 fl oz/125 ml) of milk. Let stand without stirring until gelatin is moistened, about 10 minutes.

2 Meanwhile, pour remaining 1 cup (8 fl oz/250 ml) milk into a small saucepan over medium heat. If using a vanilla bean, scrape seeds from vanilla halves into milk, then add empty bean pod. (If using vanilla extract, add it with yogurt, below.) Add granulated sugar, bring mixture to a gentle simmer, and cook, stirring, just until sugar is dissolved. Remove from heat.

3 Add gelatin mixture to pan and stir until gelatin is dissolved, 3–5 minutes. Pour into a large bowl. Let cool to lukewarm, about 10 minutes. Remove vanilla pod. Add yogurt (and vanilla extract, if using) and stir until blended.

4 Lightly brush insides of six 6-oz (185-g) ramekins with oil and arrange on a rimmed baking sheet. Divide yogurt mixture evenly among prepared ramekins. Cover and refrigerate until set, at least 8 hours or up to 2 days.

5 Just before serving, in a bowl, toss berries with brown sugar and vinegar. To serve, gently run a knife between panna cotta and sides of ramekins to loosen. Invert a dessert plate over ramekin and, holding plate and ramekin together, turn over and remove ramekin. If panna cotta doesn't slip out easily, dip bottoms of ramekins in warm water for a few seconds and dry before inverting again. Spoon berries evenly around each panna cotta, drizzling plate with juices. Serve right away.

Creamy vanilla frozen yogurt is divine with this sweet cherry compote. You can serve the compote warm or chilled, and it can be made a day ahead. A cherry pitter is handy, but not necessary; simply halve the cherries and remove the pits over a bowl to catch any drips.

CHERRY COMPOTE WITH VANILLA FROZEN YOGURT

ripe fresh cherries, 2 lb (1 kg), stemmed and pitted
sugar, ⅓ cup (3 oz/90 g)
fresh orange juice, ⅓ cup (3 fl oz/80 ml)
fresh lemon juice, 2 Tbsp
vanilla bean, 1, split lengthwise
vanilla low-fat frozen yogurt, 1½ pints (24 oz/750 g), slightly softened

MAKES 6 SERVINGS

1 In a saucepan over medium-high heat, stir together cherries, sugar, and orange and lemon juices.

2 Using tip of a small sharp knife, scrape seeds from vanilla bean halves into pan. Cook, stirring often, until cherries begin to release their juices and sugar is dissolved, about 3 minutes. Adjust heat to maintain a gentle simmer and cook, stirring occasionally, until cherries are soft but still hold their shape, 6–8 minutes longer.

3 To serve, scoop frozen yogurt into bowls or dessert glasses and spoon cherries on top. Serve right away.

Here's an elegant and healthy take on an ice-cream sundae. Feel free to swap in chocolate frozen yogurt for the vanilla.

cherries
- Known to reduce the risk of heart disease, diabetes, and some cancers
- Rich in melatonin, which helps regulate sleep
- Source of antioxidants

per serving 330 calories, 11 g protein, 70 g carbs, 3 g fat (1 g saturated fat), 45 mg cholesterol, 3 g fiber, 45 mg sodium

A handful of simple ingredients, including almonds and olive oil, come together to make this exceptional, not-too-sweet cake. Garnish it with any pretty fresh fruit you like, or serve it plain—it will still be delicious. Make sure you have a springform pan before getting started.

OLIVE OIL—ALMOND CAKE

This out-of-the-ordinary cake, rich in "good" fats and other nutrients, is a great recipe to keep in mind for the occasional indulgence.

olive oil
- Extremely rich in heart-healthy monounsaturated fats
- Rich in unique polyphenols that prevent cancer and stomach ulcers

almonds
- One of nature's richest sources of vitamin E
- Contain prebiotics, compounds that promote digestive health
- Promote heart health and lower cholesterol

per serving 250 calories, 5 g protein, 34 g carbs, 11 g fat (2 g saturated fat), 50 mg cholesterol, 2 g fiber, 200 mg sodium

unsalted butter, 2 tsp

all-purpose flour, for dusting, plus 1½ cups (7½ oz/235 g)

baking powder, 2 tsp

salt, ½ tsp

blanched almonds, ½ cup (2½ oz/75 g) coarsely chopped

sugar, 1 cup (8 oz/250 g)

eggs, 3 large

olive oil, ⅓ cup (3 fl oz/80 ml)

orange zest, 1 Tbsp minced

pure vanilla extract, 2 tsp

orange, 1 large, peeled and thinly sliced

fresh pomegranate seeds, 2 Tbsp

honey, 1 Tbsp

MAKES 12 SERVINGS

1 Preheat oven to 350°F (180°C). Butter a 9-inch (23-cm) springform pan. Dust with flour and shake out excess.

2 In a bowl, stir together flour, baking powder, and salt. In a food processor, combine nuts and ¼ cup (2 oz/60 g) of sugar and process until finely ground. Add to bowl with flour mixture and combine.

3 In a bowl, using an electric mixer set on medium-high speed, beat eggs together until frothy. Add remaining ¾ cup (6 oz/185 g) sugar and beat on high speed until thick and pale yellow, 6–8 minutes. On low speed, beat in olive oil, orange zest, and vanilla. Using a rubber spatula, gently fold flour-almond mixture into egg mixture until well blended. Scrape batter into prepared pan.

4 Bake cake until top is golden brown and a skewer inserted into center comes out clean, about 30 minutes. Let cool in pan on a wire rack for 10 minutes. Run a thin-bladed knife around edge of pan to loosen sides of cake, and remove pan sides. Let cool completely.

5 Before serving, top cake with orange slices and pomegranate seeds and drizzle with honey. Cut into wedges and serve.

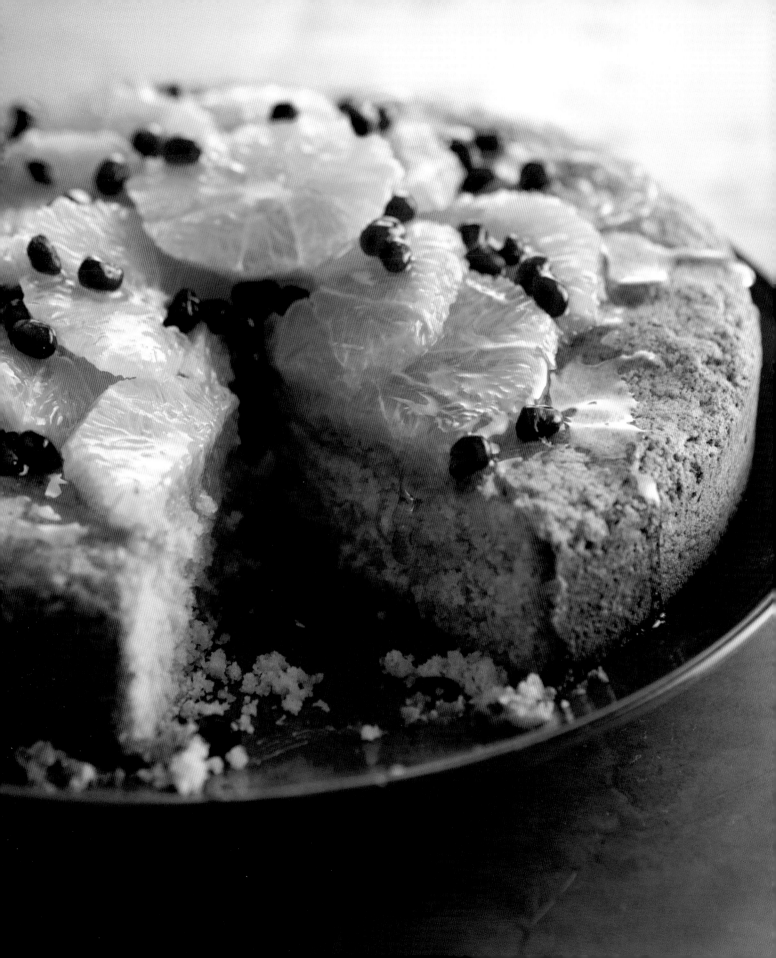

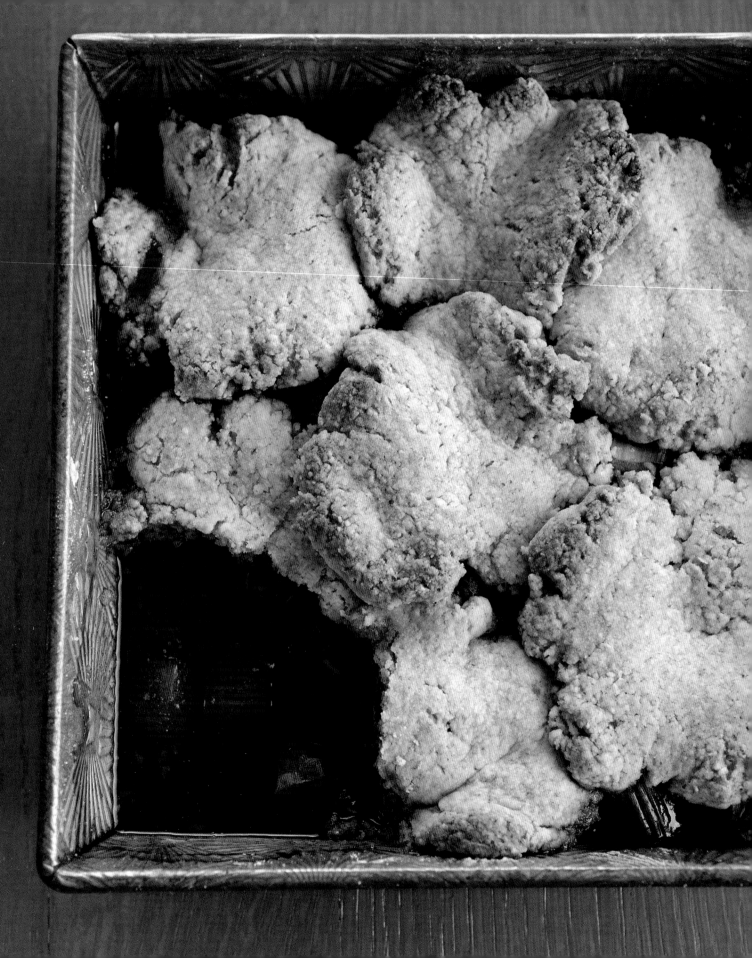

This rustic dessert has a flaky, nutty, biscuitlike topping and lots of sweet, juicy fruit. Look for rhubarb, an edible plant, in the markets during spring and summer months. Be sure to trim away and discard any green parts before using.

RASPBERRY–RHUBARB PANDOWDY

FOR TOPPING

pecans, ½ cup (3 oz/90 g)

rolled oats, ¾ cup (2¼ oz/67 g)

all-purpose flour, 1 cup (5 oz/155 g)

light brown sugar, ¼ cup firmly packed (2 oz/60 g)

baking powder, 2 tsp

salt, ¼ tsp

unsalted butter, 6 Tbsp (3 oz/90 g), cut into chunks

low-fat (2%) milk, ⅓–½ cup (3–4 fl oz/80–125 ml)

FOR FILLING

granulated sugar, ⅓ cup (3 oz/90 g)

cornstarch, 1 Tbsp

raspberries, 4 cups (1 lb/500 g)

rhubarb, 1 lb (500 g), cut into slices about ½ inch (12 mm) thick (about 3 cups)

MAKES 10 SERVINGS

1 Preheat oven to 375°F (190°C). Spread pecans in a single layer on a baking sheet and toast in oven until lightly browned, 5–8 minutes. Remove from oven and let cool slightly, then chop coarsely and set aside. Leave oven on.

2 To make topping, in a food processor, whirl oats until finely ground. Add flour, brown sugar, baking powder, salt, and toasted pecans and pulse to combine. Add butter and pulse until the mixture forms coarse, uniform crumbs. Add milk slowly through food tube, pulsing just until mixture starts to come together into a soft dough. Remove blade from food processor.

3 To make filling, in a large bowl, whisk together granulated sugar and cornstarch. Add fruit and toss to coat. Scrape into an 8-inch (20-cm) square baking dish or other shallow 2–3-qt (2–3-l) baking dish and smooth top.

4 Using lightly floured hands, pick up small handfuls of dough, pat into flat rounds about ⅓ inch (9 mm) thick, and arrange over fruit.

5 Bake until topping is golden brown and juices are bubbling, 30–35 minutes. Transfer to a wire rack and, using back of a spoon, break up the topping a little and push it down into bubbling juices. Let cool for at least 10 minutes before serving. Serve warm or at room temperature.

In this recipe, fresh fruit, whole grains, and nuts mingle in a sensible dessert that won't derail a healthy eating plan.

raspberries
- Outstanding source of fiber
- Loaded with vitamin C
- Rich in phytochemicals that protect against cancer

pecans
- High in vitamin E, which promotes a healthy immune system
- Contain nearly 20 different vitamins and minerals

per serving 280 calories, 5 g protein, 40 g carbs, 12 g fat (5 g saturated fat), 20 mg cholesterol, 6 g fiber, 140 mg sodium

Both rolled oats and whole-wheat flour give a rustic texture to these chocolate-studded dessert bars, reminiscent of oatmeal–chocolate chip cookies. Long and slender, they are perfectly shaped for dipping into a tall glass of nonfat milk.

DARK CHOCOLATE OATMEAL BARS

If you're baking for someone with a nut allergy, or want to decrease the amount of fat in the recipe, substitute dried fruits, such as cherries or cranberries, for the walnuts.

oats
- Rich in beta-glucan, shown to lower cholesterol
- Excellent source of zinc, iron, and magnesium
- Source of antioxidants linked to cardiovascular health

per bar 220 calories, 4 g protein, 27 g carbs, 12 g fat (6 g saturated fat), 40 mg cholesterol, 2 g fiber, 95 mg sodium

unsalted butter, 2 tsp, plus ¾ cup (6 oz/185 g), at room temperature

walnut pieces, 1 cup (4 oz/125 g)

all-purpose flour, ¾ cup (4 oz/125 g)

whole-wheat flour, ¾ cup (4 oz/125 g)

rolled oats, 1 cup (3 oz/90 g)

baking powder, 1½ tsp

salt, ½ tsp

light brown sugar, 1¼ cups firmly packed (9 oz/280 g)

large eggs, 3

pure vanilla extract, 1 Tbsp

bittersweet chocolate, 6 oz (185 g), chopped

MAKES 24 BARS

1 Preheat oven to 350°F (180°C). Line a 9-by-13-inch (23-by-33-cm) baking dish with aluminum foil and lightly grease foil with 2 teaspoons butter. Spread walnuts in a single layer on a baking sheet and toast in oven until lightly browned, about 10 minutes. Remove from oven and let cool slightly, then chop coarsely and set aside. Leave oven on.

2 In a large bowl, stir together flours, oats, baking powder, and salt; set aside.

3 In another large bowl or bowl of an electric mixer, beat ¾ cup butter and brown sugar until light and well blended. Beat in eggs, one at a time, scraping down sides of bowl as needed. Beat in vanilla.

4 Add flour mixture to wet ingredients and stir with a wooden spoon or beat on low speed with an electric mixer until just combined. Stir in chocolate and walnuts.

5 Spread batter evenly in prepared baking dish. Bake until top is golden brown and a wooden skewer inserted into center comes out with moist crumbs attached, about 35 minutes. Let cool completely in pan, then use edges of foil to lift bar out of pan onto a cutting board. Cut into 24 bars. Serve at once, or store in an airtight container at room temperature for up to 3 days.

Once you've tasted homemade chocolate pudding—and discovered how simple it is to prepare—you'll never consider instant again. This version has the flavors of Mexican chocolate, imbued with cinnamon and just a hint of heat from cayenne.

MEXICAN CHOCOLATE PUDDING

light brown sugar, ¼ cup firmly packed (2 oz/60 g)

cornstarch, 2 Tbsp

ground cinnamon, ½ tsp

cayenne pepper, ⅛ tsp

salt, ⅛ tsp

low-fat (2%) milk, 2 cups (16 fl oz/500 ml)

large egg yolks, 2

bittersweet chocolate, 4 oz (125 g), finely chopped

pure vanilla extract, ½ tsp

MAKES 6 SERVINGS

1 In a small bowl, stir together brown sugar, cornstarch, cinnamon, cayenne, and salt. Set aside.

2 In a saucepan, whisk together milk and egg yolks. Add brown sugar mixture and whisk to mix well. Bring to a simmer over medium heat, stirring constantly with a heatproof rubber spatula or a wooden spoon until sugar is dissolved and mixture begins to bubble around edges of pot, about 5 minutes. Cook gently, stirring constantly, for 1 minute longer, then remove from heat. Stir in chocolate until melted and smooth, followed by vanilla.

3 Spoon pudding into 6 ramekins or dessert glasses, dividing it evenly, and smooth tops. Place a piece of waxed paper directly on surface of each serving to prevent a skin from forming. Refrigerate until well chilled, about 2 hours. Serve cold.

This homemade pudding is a healthy alternative to high-fat chocolate ice cream, and the creamy texture is deceiving.

cinnamon
- Helps balance blood sugar
- Rich in manganese, a mineral needed for a healthy metabolism
- Prevents blood clots, improving heart health

per serving 200 calories, 5 g protein, 28 g carbs, 9 g fat (5 g saturated fat), 70 mg cholesterol, 1 g fiber, 105 mg sodium

Keeping a good supply of pantry staples on hand will provide a solid foundation for putting together quick meals throughout the week. If your cupboard is well stocked, you should only need to shop a couple of times a week for perishable ingredients.

HEALTHY PANTRY STAPLES

ORGANIZING YOUR PANTRY

Nonperishable foods can easily get lost in the recesses of dark cupboards, so don't neglect these areas of your kitchen.

label Always write the purchase date on foods you buy in bulk, as well as on other items that lose freshness quickly, like baking powder and spices.

store Heat and sunlight will shorten the life of your dried and bottled goods, so find cool, dark places to store these items (not next to your stove). Consider storing bulk items like flour, grains, pasta, and beans in airtight jars or containers.

rotate Regularly take stock of what's in your pantry, rotating older items to the front and moving newer items to the back. Discard items that have passed their expiration date, and make a list of items that you need to replace.

CANNED & JARRED GOODS
- ✓ albacore tuna and/or wild salmon, packed in water
- ✓ low-sodium beans (black, white, pinto, and/or chickpeas)
- ✓ low-sodium broth (chicken, beef, and/or vegetable)
- ✓ low-sodium crushed or diced tomatoes
- ✓ olives
- ✓ roasted red bell peppers

DRIED PASTA, GRAINS & LEGUMES
- ✓ brown rice
- ✓ buckwheat noodles
- ✓ bulgur wheat (quick-cooking)
- ✓ *farro* (semi-pearled)
- ✓ lentils
- ✓ quinoa
- ✓ rolled oats
- ✓ whole-wheat couscous
- ✓ whole-wheat pasta

OILS & VINEGARS
- ✓ canola, peanut, or grapeseed oil
- ✓ olive oil (regular and extra-virgin)
- ✓ sesame oil (toasted)
- ✓ balsamic vinegar
- ✓ rice wine vinegar
- ✓ white or red wine vinegar

OTHER FLAVORINGS
- ✓ agave nectar
- ✓ Asian chile sauce
- ✓ capers
- ✓ Dijon mustard
- ✓ honey
- ✓ hot-pepper sauce
- ✓ low-sodium soy sauce
- ✓ maple syrup
- ✓ sea salt and kosher salt
- ✓ spices and dried herbs
- ✓ tomato paste (tube)

BAKING & MISC
- ✓ baking powder
- ✓ baking soda
- ✓ all-purpose, unbleached flour
- ✓ buckwheat flour
- ✓ whole-wheat flour
- ✓ dried fruit
- ✓ nuts and seeds
- ✓ brown sugar
- ✓ granulated sugar

FRESH FOODS
- ✓ garlic
- ✓ onions
- ✓ shallots

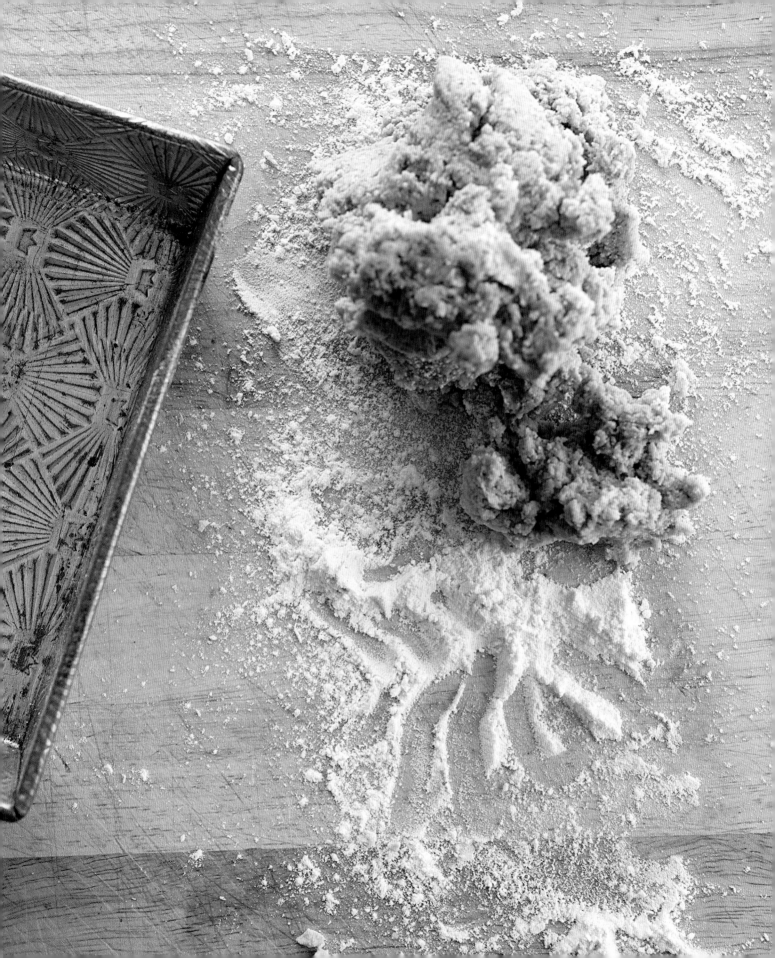

When you're focusing on simple meals that highlight fresh ingredients, it's important that those ingredients taste great. In-season produce is more flavorful, and more nutritious, than produce that's been shipped long distances to reach your grocery store.

SEASONAL FRUITS & VEGETABLES

KEEP ORGANIC IN MIND
If you're not sure where you stand on organic produce, you're not alone. Stay informed so you'll know what to reach for in the produce aisle.

check the label In the United States, the selling of organic produce is tightly controlled and regulated. When you see the certified organic label on produce, you can be assured that farmers have followed guidelines regarding the use of harmful chemicals.

prioritize purchases Organic produce can be expensive. If you want to prioritize what you buy, check out the Environmental Working Group's annual produce shopping guide (ewg.org), which lists fruits and vegetables with the highest pesticide levels. Chart toppers include apples, celery, lettuce, nectarines, peaches, potatoes, spinach, strawberries, and red bell peppers.

FRUITS	spring	summer	fall	winter
apples			X	X
apricots		X		
blackberries		X	X	
blood oranges	X		X	
blueberries	X	X		
cherries	X	X		
cranberries			X	X
grapefruits				X
lemons	X			X
limes		X	X	
mandarins	X			X
Meyer lemons	X			X
melons (cantaloupe, honeydew, watermelon)		X		
nectarines		X		
oranges	X			X
peaches		X		
pears			X	X
plums		X		
pluots		X		
pomegranates			X	X
raspberries	X	X	X	
rhubarb	X	X		
strawberries	X	X		
tangerines	X			X

VEGETABLES	spring	summer	fall	winter
artichokes	X		X	X
arugula	X	X	X	
asparagus	X			
avocados	X	X	X	
beets		X	X	
bell peppers		X		
broccoli	X		X	X
broccoli rabe			X	X
Brussels sprouts			X	X
cabbage			X	X
carrots	X			X
cauliflower		X	X	X
chard			X	X
cucumbers		X		
eggplants		X		
English peas	X			
fennel			X	X
green beans		X		
green onions	X	X	X	X
kale			X	X
leeks	X		X	
mushrooms	X		X	
onions		X		
radishes	X	X	X	
romaine lettuce				X
snow peas	X	X		
spinach	X		X	
sugar snap peas	X	X		
sweet corn		X		
sweet potatoes			X	X
tomatoes		X	X	
watercress	X		X	
winter squash			X	X
zucchini and other summer squash		X		

HEALTHY COOKING TIPS

Here are a few easy ways to curb salt and fat at the store and in the kitchen.

compare cans Packaged and canned foods like broth, tomatoes, and beans can be high in sodium and other unhealthy ingredients. Find a quality brand that offers low-sodium versions of these foods. Remember to drain and rinse canned beans to reduce their sodium content by up to 40 percent.

keep it slim Use nonfat or 1 percent milk and yogurt, and reduced-fat versions of cheese and sour cream whenever possible.

taste and measure Taste food before salting it, and look to other seasonings like citrus juice, herbs, and spices to boost flavor, as well. Always measure salt and oil instead of pouring it directly from the container.

BASIC RECIPES

COOKED DRIED BEANS

Pick over dried beans and discard any misshapen beans or stones, then rinse under cold running water and drain. Place in a large bowl with cold water to cover by a few inches and let soak for at least 4 hours or up to overnight. Drain the beans, place in a saucepan with water to cover by about 4 inches (10 cm), and bring to a boil over high heat. Reduce the heat to low, cover partially, and simmer until the beans are tender but not mushy, 1–3 hours, depending on the variety and age of the beans (test them often for doneness). Season lightly with salt. Serve warm, or let the beans cool completely in their cooking liquid, then drain and store in an airtight container in the refrigerator for up to 3 days or in a heavy-duty zippered plastic bag in the freezer for up to 3 months.

SOAKED BULGUR

Put 1 part bulgur in a heatproof bowl. Pour an equal part boiling water over the bulgur, cover the bowl tightly with aluminum foil, and let stand for 30 minutes. Drain any remaining water from the bulgur and fluff with a fork before serving.

COOKED QUINOA

Bring 2 parts water or broth to a boil in a saucepan over high heat. Add 1 part quinoa, well rinsed in a colander, to the pan and reduce the heat to low. Cover and simmer until the grains are tender and the water is absorbed, about 15 minutes. Let cool slightly before serving.

COOKED BROWN RICE

Combine 2 parts water, 1 part brown rice, and a generous pinch of salt in a saucepan over high heat and bring to a boil. Reduce the heat to low, cover, and simmer gently until the water is absorbed, 40–45 minutes. Serve warm, or let cool and store in an airtight container or zippered plastic bags in the refrigerator for up to 3 days or in the freezer for up to 3 months.

POACHED OR SAUTÉED CHICKEN BREAST

To poach: Bring a large saucepan of water to a boil over high heat. Add ½ teaspoon salt and 2 or 3 boneless, skinless chicken breast halves. Reduce the heat until the water is barely simmering and cook until the chicken is just opaque in the center, 8–10 minutes. *To sauté:* Season both sides of each chicken breast half with salt and pepper. In a frying pan, heat a thin film of canola or olive oil over medium heat. Add the chicken and cook, turning once, until opaque in the center, 4–5 minutes per side. Serve, or let cool and store in an airtight container in the refrigerator for up to 4 days.

POACHED SALMON

Bring a large saucepan of water to a boil over high heat. Add ¼ teaspoon salt, 1 thick slice yellow onion, 2 lemon slices, and 2 or 3 skinned salmon fillets. Reduce the heat until the water is barely simmering and cook until the salmon is just opaque in the center, about 10 minutes per inch (2.5 cm) of thickness. Serve, or let cool and store in an airtight container in the refrigerator for up to 2 days.

HARD-BOILED EGGS

Put eggs in a saucepan and add cold water to cover. Place over high heat and bring the water to a boil. Reduce the heat to medium-low and simmer the eggs for 12 minutes. Place the saucepan in the sink and run cold water over the eggs to cool them. Roll each egg on a work surface to crack the shell before peeling it off. If storing for later use, leave the shell on and refrigerate for up to 1 week.

ROASTED RED PEPPERS

Place 2 red bell peppers on a rimmed baking sheet and broil, turning occasionally, until the skins are blistered and the peppers are soft, 10–15 minutes. Transfer the peppers to a paper bag to cool. Remove the skins, cut the peppers in half lengthwise, and remove the seeds and membranes. Slice into strips.

ROASTED BEETS

Preheat the oven to 400°F (200°C). Cut off any beet greens, leaving 1 inch (2.5 cm) of the stems intact; do not peel the beets. Wrap each beet in a piece of aluminum foil and place in a roasting pan. Roast until tender when pierced, about 1 hour. Let cool, then unwrap and remove the skins with your fingers.

BLANCHED VEGETABLES

Bring a saucepan of water to a boil over high heat, and prepare a bowl of ice water. When the water comes to a boil, add fresh or frozen vegetables and cook just until crisp-tender (if fresh) or just until warmed through (if frozen), 3–5 minutes. Drain the vegetables and then immediately transfer them to the ice water to stop the cooking. Drain again.

VEGETABLE STOCK

In a stockpot, combine 3 leeks, trimmed, rinsed, and cut into chunks; 2 yellow onions, coarsely chopped; 4 carrots, coarsely chopped; 3 celery stalks with leaves, chopped; 6 sprigs fresh flat-leaf parsley; 2 sprigs fresh thyme; and ¼ teaspoon peppercorns. Add about 2 qt (2 l) water and bring to a boil over high heat. Reduce the heat to medium-low, cover partially, and simmer until the vegetables are very soft and the flavors have blended, about 1 hour. Remove from the heat and strain the stock through a colander set over a large heatproof bowl. Press down on the solids to extract the liquid, and discard the solids. Use the stock at once, or let cool, cover, and refrigerate for up to 3 days or freeze for up to 3 months.

PESTO

Combine 1 cup (1 oz/30 g) tightly packed fresh basil leaves; 1 clove garlic; ¼ cup (2 fl oz/60 ml) olive oil; 2 tablespoons toasted pine nuts; ¼ teaspoon salt; and several grindings of pepper in a blender or food processor. Whirl ingredients until a coarse paste forms.

Stir in ⅓ cup (1½ oz/45 g) freshly grated Parmesan cheese. Store in an airtight container in the refrigerator for up to 4 days or in the freezer for up to 3 months.

APPLESAUCE

Peel, core, and chop 2 lb (1 kg) tart apples. Place in a large saucepan with 3 tablespoons light brown sugar, ¼ cup (2 fl oz/60 ml) water, and 1 teaspoon fresh lemon juice and stir to combine. Bring to a boil over medium-high heat, then reduce the heat to low, cover, and simmer, stirring occasionally with a wooden spoon, until the sauce is thick and slightly chunky, about 20 minutes. Taste and adjust the flavorings, adding more sugar or lemon juice if needed. Serve warm, or let cool and store in an airtight container in the refrigerator for up to 3 days or in the freezer for up to 4 months.

TOMATO SAUCE

In a large saucepan over medium-low heat, warm 2 tablespoons olive oil. Add 2 cloves garlic, pressed or minced, and sauté until fragrant, about 3 minutes. Stir in ¼ cup (2 oz/60 g) tomato paste; 1 can (28 oz/875 g) low-sodium whole plum tomatoes, roughly chopped, with juice; 5 fresh basil leaves; and ¼ teaspoon salt. Bring to a simmer and cook, stirring occasionally, until the tomatoes break down, 15–20 minutes. Using an immersion blender, process the sauce until smooth. (Or, transfer the sauce to a food processor and process until smooth.) Let cool and store in an airtight container in the refrigerator for up to 3 days or in the freezer for up to 3 months.

BASIC VINAIGRETTE

In a jar with a tight-fitting lid, combine 2 tablespoons red or white wine vinegar, 2 teaspoons Dijon mustard, and ½ teaspoon salt. Add ¼ cup (2 fl oz/60 ml) extra-virgin olive oil, cover, and shake to combine. Season with freshly ground pepper. Adjust the flavorings by using fresh lemon juice or balsamic vinegar, or adding minced garlic or herbs.

NUTRITION TERMS GLOSSARY

ANTIOXIDANTS

Antioxidants protect against and repair daily damage to our cells and tissues. They have also been linked to heart health and cancer prevention. Some come in the form of vitamins, such as vitamins C and E. Others are compounds found in plant foods such as phytonutrients like lycopene and beta-carotene, or polyphenols such as ellagic acid. The best sources of antioxidants are colorful fruits, vegetables, nuts, and whole grains.

CARBOHYDRATES

There are three main kinds of carbohydrates: starch, sugar, and fiber. Starch and sugar provide our bodies and brains with energy. Although our bodies can't digest fiber, it provides a number of significant benefits. The healthiest sources of carbohydrates are fruits, vegetables, beans, and whole grains such as whole-wheat bread and pasta, brown rice, and quinoa.

CAROTENOIDS

Carotenoids are colored pigments in plants that provide multiple health benefits such as improved vision, enhanced immunity, or protection against cancer. While beta-carotene, the pigment that gives carrots their orange color, is perhaps the most well known carotenoid, others include lycopene from tomatoes and zeaxanthin and lutein from spinach.

CHOLESTEROL

Foods from animal sources such as eggs, milk, cheese, and meat contain cholesterol, but the human body makes its own supply as well. While cholesterol in our diets was once thought to be a major contributor to high cholesterol levels, we now know that foods rich in saturated fat raise unhealthy LDL cholesterol in our blood streams more substantially than cholesterol from other food. Plant compounds like phytosterols in wheat germ, peanuts, and almonds and beta-glucan from oats have been shown to lower cholesterol.

FATS

Our bodies need fat to absorb certain vitamins, build the membranes that line our cells, and cushion our joints and organs. But fats aren't all created equal. Saturated and hydrogenated fat are linked to chronic ailments such as heart disease, while unsaturated fats can be more healthful.

monounsaturated fats Found in nuts, avocados, olive oil, and canola oil, these fats are less likely to raise levels of unhealthy LDL cholesterol, linked to heart attack and stroke. They also help keep arteries clear by maintaining levels of healthy HDL cholesterol.

polyunsaturated fats These fats can play an important role in helping control cholesterol. While most of us get plenty of the polyunsaturated fat linolenic acid from vegetable, corn, and soybean oil, our diets don't usually contain enough of heart-healthy omega-3 fats. These are found as EPA and DHA in fish or in the form of alpha linolenic acid in flaxseed, canola oil, and walnuts.

saturated fats Found in meats, dairy products, and tropical oils such as coconut oil and palm oil, these fats raise blood levels of unhealthy LDL cholesterol.

trans fats Present in hydrogenated vegetable oils in many processed and fried foods, trans fats may be even more harmful than saturated fats.

FIBER

Fiber is the component of plant foods that our bodies can't digest. Insoluble fiber does not dissolve in water and is known for preventing constipation. Soluble fiber softens in water and helps lower blood cholesterol levels. Fiber-rich diets have been linked with improved digestive health and reduced risk for type 2 diabetes and heart disease.

FLAVONOIDS

These plant compounds help prevent heart disease and possibly cancer. They include quercetin from onions and apples, anthocyanidins from berries, and isoflavones from soy.

MINERALS

Minerals are elements that our bodies need for survival. Major minerals, such as calcium, are required in larger amounts, while trace minerals like iron and zinc are needed in smaller amounts.

calcium Vital for bone health, calcium is also important for muscle contraction and blood pressure regulation. Calcium-rich foods include low-fat milk, fish with bones, and certain leafy greens such as broccoli and bok choy.

copper This trace mineral is essential for proper iron metabolism. It is also involved in wound healing and metabolism.

iron Iron helps the body transport and use oxygen, and also plays a role in immune function, cognitive development, temperature regulation, and energy metabolism.

manganese This trace mineral is needed for proper metabolism of carbohydrates, fats, and proteins. It also keeps bones and teeth healthy.

phosphorus Phosphorus helps build strong bones and teeth, aids metabolic function, and helps the body get energy from food.

potassium Potassium helps the body maintain water and mineral balance, and regulates heartbeat and blood pressure.

selenium This trace mineral works with vitamin E as an antioxidant to protect cells from damage, and also boosts immune function.

zinc Zinc promotes a healthy immune system and is critical for proper blood clotting, thyroid function, and optimal growth and reproduction.

PROTEIN

Made of amino acids, protein provides the building blocks our bodies need to synthesize cells, tissues, hormones, and antibodies. It is found in foods of animal and vegetable origin, although animal proteins contain more of the amino acids our bodies need to synthesize protein. Choose lean protein sources like fish, poultry, and legumes.

VITAMINS

Our bodies require vitamins in order to function properly. They fall into two categories: fat-soluble vitamins, which require fat for absorption and are stored in our body's fat tissue, and water-soluble vitamins, which cannot be stored and must be replenished often.

vitamin A Found in dairy products, yellow-orange fruits and vegetables, and dark green leafy vegetables, vitamin A promotes healthy skin, hair, bones, and vision. It also works as an antioxidant.

B vitamins This group of water-soluble vitamins can be found in a range of fruits and vegetables, whole grains, and dairy and meat products and includes vitamins B6 and B12, biotin, niacin, pantothenic acid, thiamin, folate, and riboflavin. Each one plays a vital role in bodily functions, including regulating metabolism and energy production, keeping the nerves and muscles healthy, and protecting against birth defects and heart disease.

vitamin C This water-soluble vitamin helps build body tissues, fights infection, helps keep gums healthy, and helps the body absorb iron. It also works as an antioxidant. It can be found in many fruits and vegetables, especially citrus fruits.

vitamin D Instrumental in building and maintaining healthy bones and teeth, vitamin D can be found in fish such as salmon and sardines, as well as in fortified milk and cereal.

vitamin E Found in nuts and seeds, whole grains, dark green vegetables, and beans, vitamin E helps form red blood cells, prevents oxidation of LDL cholesterol, and improves immunity. It also works as an antioxidant.

vitamin K Necessary for protein synthesis as well as blood clotting, vitamin K can be found in dark green vegetables, asparagus, and cabbage.

INDEX

weldonowen

415 Jackson Street, Suite 200, San Francisco, CA 94111
Telephone: 415 291 0100 Fax: 415 291 8841
www.wopublishing.com

HEALTHY IN A HURRY

Conceived and produced by Weldon Owen, Inc.
in collaboration with Williams-Sonoma, Inc.
3250 Van Ness Avenue, San Francisco, CA 94109

A WELDON OWEN PRODUCTION

Copyright © 2012 Weldon Owen, Inc. and Williams-Sonoma, Inc.
All rights reserved, including the right of reproduction
in whole or in part in any form.

Printed and bound in China
by Toppan-Leefung

First printed in 2012
10 9 8 7 6

Library of Congress control number: 2011937899

ISBN-13: 978-1-61628-213-4
ISBN-10: 1-61628-213-4

Weldon Owen is a division of
BONNIER

WELDON OWEN, INC.

CEO and President Terry Newell
VP, Sales and Marketing Amy Kaneko
Director of Finance Mark Perrigo

VP and Publisher Hannah Rahill
Executive Editor Jennifer Newens
Associate Editor Julia Nelson

Creative Director Emma Boys
Art Director Alexandra Zeigler
Senior Designer Ashley Lima

Production Director Chris Hemesath
Production Manager Michelle Duggan

Photographer Maren Caruso
Food Stylist Kim Kissling
Prop Stylist Christine Wolheim

ACKNOWLEDGMENTS

Weldon Owen wishes to thank the following people for their generous support in producing this book: Amanda Anselmino,
Carrie Bradley Neves, Ken DellaPenta, Sean Franzen, Cathy Lee, Lesli J. Neilson, Dawn Pavli, and Abby Stolfo.

NOTE ON NUTRITIONAL ANALYSIS

The numbers for all nutritional values have been rounded using the guidelines for reporting nutrient levels on U.S. food labels.
If you have particular concerns about any nutrient needs, consult a doctor or registered dietitian.